Also by Anne Rogers

Experiencing Psychiatry (with Ron Lacey and David Pilgrim)

A Sociology of Mental Health and Illness (with David Pilgrim)

Demanding Patients? Analysing the Use of Primary Care (with Karen Hassell and Gerry Nicolaas)

Also by David Pilgrim

Experiencing Psychiatry (with Ron Lacey and Anne Rogers)

A Sociology of Mental Health Illness (with Anne Rogers)

Psychotherapy and Society

Clinical Psychology Observed (with Andy Treacher)

Mental Health Policy in Britain

Second Edition

Anne Rogers

and

David Pilgrim

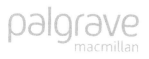

First edition 1996
Second edition 2001

Published by
PALGRAVE MACMILLAN
Houndmills, Basingstoke, Hampshire RG21 6XS and
175 Fifth Avenue, New York, N. Y. 10010
Companies and representatives throughout the world

PALGRAVE MACMILLAN is the global academic imprint of the Palgrave Macmillan division of St. Martin's Press, LLC and of Palgrave Macmillan Ltd. Macmillan® is a registered trademark in the United States, United Kingdom and other countries. Palgrave is a registered trademark in the European Union and other countries.

ISBN 0–333–94792–4 hardback
ISBN 0–333–94793–2 paperback

This book is printed on paper suitable for recycling and made from fully managed and sustained forest sources.

A catalogue record for this book is available from the British Library.

Library of Congress Cataloging-in-Publication Data

Rogers, Anne.
    Mental health policy in Britain / Anne Rogers and David Prilgrim. –2nd ed.
        p. cm.
    Includes bibliographical references and index.
    ISBN 0–333–94792–4
    1. Mental health policy–Great Britain. 2. Mental health policy–Great Britain–History. 3. Mental health services–Great Britain. 4. Mental health services–Great Britain–History.   I. Pilgrim, David, 1950–   II. Title.

RA790.7.G7 R645 2000
362.2'0941–dc21   00–048335

11   10   9   8   7   6   5   4
11   10   09   08   07   06   05   04

Printed in China

Contents

List of Figures and Tables

Figures

Tables

Preface to the Second Edition

There are two main ways of approaching the question of policy formation. The first is to examine statements of *intent* about policy. The second is to examine policy as the *outcome of a process* of implementation (Allsop, 1984). Both of these are relevant to the mental health field. In this book we do, where relevant, take the statements made by government and other agencies as a benchmark for examining particular issues (e.g., in relation to mental health legislation). However, this is given less salience than 'the policy-as-process' focus, which looks to the actions of groups of actors to explain the actual implementation of policy and the configuration of service provision in particular local contexts.

We take this process approach because policy formation is not as centralised as it sometimes appears. It is often shaped by specific local factors and the actions of the social actors who provide, manage or receive services. This has been particularly evident in mental health policy and practice in Britain (and elsewhere) since de-institutionalisation. Compared to the centralised state mental hospital system, the latter constitutes a decentralised patchwork of services and events which are spread across a range of agencies and levels of government.

In contrast to other areas of social policy, successive British governments have been content to state the objectives of mental health policy in broad terms, leaving the rest to be interpreted and implemented by those working in different localities. The production of prescriptive official documentation has not had as much impact as the actions and agencies external to government in shaping practice and policy. Indeed, the copious number of committees and reports which have flourished are often notable for their *failure* to determine what has happened on the ground and for their vague conclusions which have tended to set low expectations of practical change. This was particularly the case in relation to practice and policy developments during the 1980s. At that time changes in mental health practice were, to a large extent, influenced by academic commentary about community care and constituted by an amalgam of disparate practices promoted by voluntary or independent organisations such as MIND, with individual localities promoting a variegated picture of new services.

It is only relatively recently – during the 1990s – that mental health policy *per se* has assumed a higher profile within the Department of Health (DH) and other government agencies. During this recent period there has been a growing emphasis on more closely specifying the content and details of what services should be delivered. Even within the wake of this more prescriptive period we are still not clear how directives are being embraced or resisted within localities by stakeholders. At the time of writing we await the impact of one of the most tightly prescriptive documents yet produced by central government (the National Service Framework for Mental Health, discussed in Chapter 12).

Our analysis in this book is biased towards the activities of stakeholders and their perspectives for another reason. There is often a tendency for those who are working as agents of government (e.g., local mental health service managers) to take the newest policy statement as the most meaningful and significant. Whilst this must be the focus of managers attempting to implement the latest government dictate, the success, failure and trajectory of mental health policy formation are determined by a broader context. Significant shifts in mental health policy and practice are not traceable to some particular committee's report of intention but emerge because of a range of formative factors and the actions of several agencies. A singular focus on social administrative detail is likely to distract us from attempts at explanation which are rooted in the context in which mental health issues are formed and policy developed.

The book is divided into three parts. The first provides a conceptual introduction to our framework for understanding mental health policy as a process. We have argued elsewhere that this is best done by drawing upon a range of disciplinary insights (Pilgrim and Rogers, 1999). The second part examines a variety of historical aspects of British mental health policy. The third part has eight chapters which reflect on: mental health professions; patients; mental health promotion; primary care; community mental health care; whether the institution has been left behind; and whether current services are effective. The final chapter, which contains a summary of the main social administrative features of current mental health policy, connects past, present and future developments.

When we were asked to provide a second edition of a book entitled *Mental Health Policy in Britain*, we were reticent about retaining the word 'Britain'. In the five years since we finished the first edition, the UK has seen the emergence of a new Parliament in Scotland and assemblies in Wales and Northern Ireland. For a good while before these events, the separate nations of the UK had sometimes produced separate guidance or law in relation to social policy. At times policy innovations were evident outside England before Westminster mimicked them: for example, a watchdog commission emerged in Scotland before England and Wales. Despite these short and long signs of devolution and fragmentation we have opted to retain 'Britain' and 'British' in the text, mainly for two reasons, one legislative and the other cultural.

Although much of this book is indeed Anglocentric, Westminster legislation has dominated, and still dominates, the UK. Where it has not had direct legal jurisdiction over the Celtic fringe, then the other nation-states have still tended to reflect similar cultural processes in professional circles. For example, the Care Programme Approach did not apply in Wales but the concern to systematise care management was evident there. Another example is in relation to the 1983 Mental Health Act. Although the Mental Health (NI) Order was passed in 1986 for Northern Ireland, which had a different emphasis about hospital admission from the English legislation, in most regards it followed the spirit and detail of the 1983 Act. As Prior (1993) notes, this was in part because non-English variants at that time were determined by a Standing Committee system, not by a full public debate in Parliament. Such a system has only very recently been superseded by the governmental arrangements devolved from London.

As for culture, the four nation states of the UK – and, for that matter, Eire – are overwhelmingly English speaking. Also the professional norms in health and social care in the British Isles have more that connects them than separates them. At the same time, as we indicated at the start of the preface, there are also parochial differences. Such differences occur across the British Isles and they may be determined by common cross-national variables. For example, the demographic and economic features of rural life may create similar conditions for the mental health of the population and service delivery in the Scottish Highlands, Snowdonia, the mountains of Mourne and the Peak District. These areas have more in common with one another than with urban localities within their own countries. We are aware that these arguments are all open to legitimate challenge. However, for now, we consider that more would be lost than gained by replacing 'Britain' with 'England', as most of the text is relevant to students of mental health policy throughout the British Isles.

ANNE ROGERS
DAVID PILGRIM

Acknowledgements

In the past few years, a number of people have influenced our thoughts about the contents of the book, or have helped us with technical aspects of the revised manuscript. Special thanks go to Pat Bracken, Peter Campbell, Alison Faulkner, Linda Gask, Catherine Gray, Pat Guinan, Brian Hoser, David Morris, Nick Morris, Steve Onyett, Steven Pilgrim, Keith Povey, Bonnie Sibbald, Geraldine Strathdee and Phil Thomas.

ANNE ROGERS
DAVID PILGRIM

List of Abbreviations

ACT	Assertive Community Treatment
ASP	anti-social personality disorder
ASW	Approved Social Worker
CAPO	Campaign for the Abolition of Psychiatry
CMHC	Community Mental Health Centre
CMHM	Community Mental Health Movement
CMHN	Community Mental Health Nurse
CMHT	Community Mental Health Team
CNS	central nervous system
COP	community-orientated primary care
CPA	Care Programme Approach
CPD	continuous professional development
CPN	community psychiatric nurse
CRU	Civil Resettlement Unit
CTO	Compulsory Treatment Order
DGH	District General Hospital
DH	Department of Health
DHSS	Department of Health and Social Security
DRGs	Diagnostic Related Groups
DSM	Diagnostic and Statistical Manual
ECT	electroconvulsive therapy
EMS	Emergency Medical Service
ERG	external reference group
FHSA	Family Health Services Authority
GP	general practitioner
GMC	General Medical Council
HAS	Health Advisory Service
HAZ	Health Action Zone
HEA	Health Education Authority
ICDIO	International Classification of Diseases
IRG	Internal Reference Group
MHAC	Mental Health Action Commission
MHF	Mental Health Foundation
MIND	National Association for Mental Health

NHS	National Health Service
NHSE	National Health Service Executive
NHSME	National Health Service Management Executive
NSF	National Service Framework
OPCS	Office of Population and Census Statistics
PCG	Primary Care Group
PCT	Primary Care Trust
RCT	Randomised Control Trial
SANE	Schizophrenia A National Emergency
SPO	structure, process, outcome
UKAN	United Kingdom Advocacy Network
UKCC	United Kingdom Central Committee
WHO	World Health Organisation

Part I

Understanding Policy Formation

1

Policy Formation and Mental Health Services

Introduction

An understanding of mental health policy requires reference to a range of interpretative frameworks. When discussing health policy in general, Palmer and Short (1989) draw attention to four major policy perspectives:

- economic
- political science
- sociological
- epidemiological and public health

Another we add later is that of *comparative social policy*. Here we will highlight the utility of each of these perspectives in illuminating mental health policy developments and processes. The purpose is not to provide a comprehensive or exhaustive account of the different perspectives or their applicability to every aspect of mental health; rather, it is to outline the different conceptualisations which can be applied to mental health policy and practice. For the purposes of analysis here we follow a traditional formulation and have isolated the different perspectives across disciplinary boundaries. However, it is important to note that there is not a set of discrete boundaries which neatly separates disciplinary trends; instead, there are sedimented layers of knowledge which overlap unevenly.

The Economic Perspective

This centres on two main concepts: supply and demand. The former refers to the quantity of a commodity that providers are willing to offer for sale at a price, and the latter refers to the quantity of the commodity that consumers are prepared to buy at a specified price. This market-focused model has limitations in relation to health care service-users in general and those using mental health services in particular. Here are some examples:

(1) Only some people with mental health problems can be described unambiguously as 'consumers'. The term applies only to those using private therapists voluntarily or who choose to use the small level of privately-funded inpatient facilities. In other words, an economic model assumes that patients are purchasers. In fact, even when they do buy therapy it is not a tangible product (like a washing machine) but an intangible expectation that their psychological well-being will be improved or their distress ameliorated.

(2) Between 1983 and 1997, with the introduction of market principles in the National Health Service (NHS), the terms 'purchaser' (or 'commissioner') and 'provider' were introduced. However, this did not mean individual patients (or individual 'shoppers') were purchasers, but referred to commissioning authorities or GP fundholders which would buy services on behalf of local groups of patients. Thus the notion of demand being linked to individual consumers in general economics did not apply to publicly provided mental health services even when market principles dominated government ideology. The notion of the NHS as a market was a misnomer: it was never more than a 'quasi-market'.

(3) In the ordinary market-place consumption takes place on the basis of choices being available. With the exception of that minority of patients rich enough to shop around for private therapists, most NHS patients have to accept what is given in their locality. Clinical professionals are monopoly suppliers of services. General practitioners (GPs) control to whom the person is referred and the specialist then determines what treatment is given. This context tends to produce services which are limited in range by the pressures of a professional monopoly of supply plus resource constraints. These twin processes militate against the individual patient having choices.

(4) The market model also has a clear definition of the client. As well as the term 'purchaser' not applying to individual patients, there is a further ambiguity about who is the client of psychiatric services. Mental patients themselves are arguably only clients when they opt to

approach services for help. But there is a variety of other circumstances in which people become mental patients. In private dwellings their relatives may ask for help with a crisis. If, subsequently, the patient is forcibly taken away and treated by psychiatric staff, then it is the relatives and not the identified patient who are the clients of psychiatry. Therefore, they, not the labelled or identified patient, are having a 'service' provided for them. Similar arguments apply to the removal of patients from a public place to a place of safety by the police for a psychiatric assessment. In these circumstances arguably the police and the complaining public, not the patient, are the clients. Whenever patienthood is imposed on a person (by involuntary detention or treatment), it is clearly nonsensical to construe them as a 'customer'.

(5) Everyday choices in the market-place entail the purchaser of goods being able to understand clearly what they want (e.g., a machine that efficiently washes their clothes). This is less clear in health services, which entail a knowledge imbalance between patients and professionals. In relation to psychiatric patients there is the additional common assumption operating around them that, due to lack of insight, they do not appreciate what they need. Thus 'need' is defined by suppliers of mental health services, whereas in the market-place it is defined by the consumer (though the latter's view can be shaped by sales talk and advertising).

Thus, the market-focused model of traditional economics can be applied only inadequately to mental health services. However, *because* the model fails to work as a basis for explaining service policy development, the contradictions it sets up (i.e., the limitations listed above) provide us with some interesting critical questions about why 'services' fail in their own terms. That is, they highlight why the term 'mental health *services*' is problematic. What evidence is there that they promote or improve mental health, as their name implies? Also, in what sense are they 'services': services to whom and to what end? In the first regard, surely it is mental illness which is being treated and not mental health facilitated. In the second regard, we can see that psychiatry has many potential clients beyond the patients it labels. It operates as much to control disruptive conduct, and bring to an end social crises, as it does to ameliorate mental distress.

However, whilst standard economic formulae about supply and demand have a limited value for policy analysis, health economists have provided rich conceptual tools for analysing the utility and effectiveness of services. There are four main economic methods of analysis in this regard:

(a) *cost-benefit* – that is, measuring how much interventions cost against the economic benefits they generate (e.g., the price of treating disability against savings on social security payments);
(b) *cost-minimisation* – that is, comparing different interventions with equal claims of efficacy to check which is the cheapest;
(c) *cost-effectiveness* – that is, extending cost-benefit analysis to look at, say, the (quantified) extension of life by an intervention;
(d) *cost-utility* – that is, extending the above to look at the improvement in quality of life for patients created by an intervention.

Each of the four forms of analysis has both strengths and weaknesses when investigating the utility and effectiveness of medical interventions with physically ill or disabled people. When the latter are *psychiatric* interventions the forms of analysis become problematic. Given the confusion about the purpose of psychiatry and whom it is serving (see above), what is to be investigated by health economists? Is it the improvement in the quality of life of patients or of their relatives? What if these are at odds with one another? What if some interventions are highly effective at suppressing disruptive conduct but have profoundly disabling and distressing effects on their recipients? Whose word is privileged about improvement following an intervention? Is it the word of the patient, or the patient's relatives, or the patient's treating professionals? When some drugs (such as anti-depressants) are cheaper than labour-intensive psychological interventions, and just as effective at reducing depressive symptoms, should the latter be abolished in favour of the former? What happens when these drugs are sometimes used for self-poisoning to commit suicide? What if some patients demand the more expensive (psychological) intervention on grounds of quality of life? In these circumstances is there a tension between cost-benefit, cost-minimisation, cost-effectiveness and cost-utility analyses?

Thus, even when a modified health economic model (which is more sophisticated than the crude market model) is utilised, it frequently does not give us simple answers to the complex questions and controversies surrounding mental health policy. However, it can provide some interesting data to contribute to those controversies. It also might clarify the relevant *questions* to ask about services and the policies generating them. One area in which a health economic perspective has proved fruitful is in assessing to what extent there are advantages and disadvantages in moving to a 'mixed economy of mental health care' in the UK. Knapp and his colleagues (1999) examined and compared the cost, quality of care and outcome implications between public and other provider sectors (e.g., NHS and voluntary sector) in a longitudinal study of people who were moved out of psychiatric hospitals in the London area. The costs of providing care were found to be lower in the private for profit sector than in the NHS-provided services. However, quality of care was found to be higher in the higher cost NHS-provided service sector.

The macro-economic perspective

Over and above the utility of economic models in the evaluation of services there is a wider 'macro' economic perspective that also needs to be taken into consideration in the field of mental health policy which extends beyond the cost-effectiveness of therapies or services. Economic analysis has a useful role in exploring how economic processes affect those who are disadvantaged or excluded because of their mental health status. Such a perspective becomes more important in an era when a greater emphasis is being placed on the wider social and economic context impacting on the mental health status of populations, and where the extent to which socio-economic utilities are maximised by those with mental health needs will significantly impact on outcomes. The argument for extending 'welfare economics' to include issues such as leisure transport and shopping (which are linked to the processes of consumption and production) are highly relevant to the quality of life of those diagnosed with a mental health problem (Cahill, 1994). So too is the extent to which secure employment opportunities are offered to those with mental health problems and the capacity of the economic system to incorporate these people into the processes of production and consumption. This fundamental political issue for contemporary mental health policy can be explored fruitfully using an economic framework of analysis, which leads us to consider the next perspective.

The Political Science Perspective

The work of political scientists forms a bridge between economic and sociological models of policy formation. Health policy analyses by Alford (1975) and Marmor (1973), focusing on the US health care system, have been generalised to other mixed economy capitalist systems: for example, in Britain (Allsop, 1984; Ham, 1985) and Australia (Palmer and Short, 1989). As with the economic analyses just discussed, the

political science perspective has relevance for understanding processes
implicating the State and its relationship with agencies and agents in
wider society. The perspective has an increasing salience in understanding the role of mental health in advanced capitalist democracies.
A political science perspective in the field of mental health policy draws
attention to the wider ideological and moral shifts within modern democracies which impact on mental health. Political processes and institutions
have important implications for the climate and development of approaches to managing mental health problems and to issues such as
the levels of inclusion or exclusion of those with mental health problems. Exemplars here are the broader political values informing service
provision and notions of citizenship in later modern welfare capitalist
states. With regard to the first of these, the principles and ideology
adopted by States have relevance to the type of mental health provision which is provided. The British legacy of the post-war settlement
of the late 1940s has meant that services have been underpinned by a
philosophy characterised by universalism. Much of this is likely to be
an enduring feature of the way in which the modern welfare state deals
with mental health problems despite a more general shift towards a
'mixed economy' of welfare. Even in more privatised systems of welfare such as the USA, mental health services have remained in large
part state-provided.

The way in which local communities perceive and interact with the
State in relation to mental health service delivery has received some
attention within a political science perspective. We move to this exploration now.

Community and identity

Despite the post-1997 fracturing of the UK, with its associated devolved government from London to the Celtic fringe, there remains a
shared *British* political culture of post-war welfarism. This remains
largely social-democratic in ideology with the concurrent presence of
aspirations for social justice alongside the injustice and oppression
inevitably present in the social processes accruing from a free market
economy. Of relevance to analysing late modern welfare provision are
the developments in the traditional academic view of citizenship in
social democracies based on concepts of individual rights, universality
and membership of a political community. There has been a renewed
interest in the notion of 'community' through the popularisation of a

communitarian philosophy, espoused by thinkers such as Etzioni (1995). This has exposed us to newly-fashioned definitions of 'community': for example, based on shared and explicit common identities, derived from race, religion, sexuality or disability. These have been added to (or, for some, have replaced) the traditional, neighbourhood-defined version of 'local' community since they cut across the traditional meanings attached to social groups such as 'family' and 'neighbourhood'.

There has also been a shift towards viewing citizenship not only as a status which people possess but as purposeful action in which individuals engage (Prior, Stewart and Walsh, 1995). There has, for example, been a growing focus on the processes involved in people formulating, giving expression to and sustaining novel collective and individual self-identities through narratives which draw upon their life experiences (Giddens, 1991). Analysis of the emergence and influence of the mental health users' movement as a new social movement embodies these conceptualisations (Rogers and Pilgrim, 1991). The demand for greater involvement and participation in the delivery of services and the rights afforded to other citizens (e.g., in employment and discrimination) has had a variable impact. Resistance, for the mental health service-users' movement, extends beyond welfare rights. The movement also insists on the recognition of the moral worth of people with mental distress and their right to be included and recognised in social relationships at different levels within social and political life. Whilst it has been argued that a defining feature of new social movements is a lack of trust in the parliamentary system, at significant points service-users may influence the form and content of democratic principles adopted by central and local government (Barnes, 1999). For example, user-representatives were included in the development of the National Service Framework for Mental Health spelling out national standards for delivering mental health services (see Chapter 12). A counter example, though, is the establishment by the current Labour government of the Social Exclusion Unit. The work of this unit has explicitly excluded any reference to mental health, and users of mental health services have been omitted from the Unit's programme of work.

Structural interests in mental health policy

The political science perspective also provides a number of models for understanding the complex processes involved in political change relevant to mental health. Alford emphasises the tensions which exist between three major structural interests in health policy. Each of these contains stakeholders who gain or lose from policy developing in this or that direction. The groupings Alford describes are described below.

1 *Professional monopolists* – mainly the medical profession and its beneficiaries such as the drug industry. This alliance would also include those members of the public persuaded by the unique authority of medicine as a profession.
2 *Corporate rationalisers* – these are planners, health administrators and some health professionals whose interests are served by greater efficiency, effectiveness and equity in health care delivery.
3 *Community interests* – these are community groups representing or being constituted by service recipients and their relatives.

The group superordinate to, and lobbied by, all three – the group with the power to make and implement policy (politicians) – is missing from Alford's model. If this fourth group were added then we can see that this framework would be a useful way of understanding the negotiations and shifts around different lobby groups: the Department of Health (DH), psychiatrists, NHS managers, users' groups and relatives' groups (these will be discussed in Chapter 2). The limitation of this model is that it works with ideal types: constructions which emphasise certain traits but which generally do not exist in this form in reality. In practice the winners and losers and roles played by discrete stakeholders are at times ambiguous and not as clear cut as implied by this theory. In particular the roles played by stakeholders in government inquiries into untoward events occurring in the community (which were made mandatory during the early 1990s) are much more ambiguous. Care centred on hospital-based mental health services provides clear cut roles and interests. By contrast, ambiguity and confusion over professional efficiency and responsibility is evident in relation to community-based care. This is particularly the case when services receive adverse attention because of untoward events such as homicides or suicides.

Marmor considers policies as political goods which are traded in a political market-place in exchange for financial backing and votes. (Note that this is an economic metaphor, not literal economics.) Marmor then emphasises that the key bargainers in this market-place are government, health care professionals and service recipients. Governments seek to provide policies which are affordable, efficient and popular in order to catch votes. What they may vary ideologically about is their position on equity. Providers seek to maximise their status and salaries.

Recipients seek to influence policies to improve their access to, choice about and experience of, services. Changes in policy and barriers to that change can be understood within this model as outcomes of power exchanges between the three key players.

One problem with this model is that it contains internal contradictions and tensions: the middle group of providers has conflicts between clinicians and bureaucrats. As we will see later in the book, the commissioning role in health services introduces a further complication to this picture, with managers and clinicians (and their interests) being present on both sides of the divide. The recipient group is ambiguous in the field of mental health because it contains some dominated by patients and some by their relatives. A second problem is that the power emphasis may not always explain why some very powerless groups can sometimes accrue apparent benefits (in terms of policy outcomes and resource allocation). In the case of psychiatric patients this might be explained by two factors: the need to allocate funds for their social subsistence and the genuine paternalistic desire on the part of other players (such as bureaucrats and politicians) to improve the lot of vulnerable and disadvantaged groups.

Within the political science paradigm a number of theories have also been influenced by Marx's concept of political economy. Scull (1977, 1979) argues that during the nineteenth century the capitalist economy necessitated the segregative control of deviant parts of the population which were disruptive or burdensome. Thus a network of workhouses, asylums and prisons emerged to contain pauper deviants. Scull goes on to argue that this segregative solution became too expensive during the second half of the twentieth century. At this point welfare capitalism entered a period of prolonged fiscal crisis. One cost-cutting policy prompted by this crisis was hospital closure ('decarceration'). Another political economy theorist, Warner, argues that fashions in psychiatric treatment have been relatively irrelevant in explaining service utilisation. Instead, he suggests that unemployment levels have been a good predictor of recovery rates for schizophrenia, with the Great Depression of the 1920s and 1930s being a period when recovery rates were at their lowest (Warner, 1985).

Sociological Perspectives

There is a range of different traditions within sociology useful to understanding mental health (Pilgrim and Rogers, 1999). For our purposes here, the relevance of social theory is that it can explain differences of both ideology and emphasis in different forms of policy analysis. The example of the differing works of Kathleen Jones and Andrew Scull is a case in point. Jones has developed a form of policy analysis which is, by her own admission, anti-theoretical (Jones, 1972, xiii) and therefore uncritically accepting of the views of dominant interest groups such as the psychiatric profession. Consequently, her work offers an account of policy development which endorses a public relations view of psychiatric history, with nineteenth-century humanitarianism (Jones, 1960, 149) and twentieth-century technical breakthroughs, such as the introduction of major tranquillisers (Jones, 1988, 82). By contrast, Scull's work (1977, 1979), based mainly on Marxian economic theory, as we have noted, offers a critical view of history and a cynical view of services.

However, sociological theories beyond the positions of Jones and Scull can also be identified. To start with Scull's Marxism, this is actually mixed with the views of Max Weber on professional dominance and social closure (Scull, 1979, 129). Weber and his followers (Freidson, 1970; Abel, 1988) place less emphasis on economics than Marxians and more of an emphasis on the negotiation of social status by different interest groups in society. Professionalisation entails some occupational groups, such as psychiatry, cornering the market and protecting their boundaries from outside intrusion and scrutiny (social closure). In doing so, this allows professionals to exert power over their clients who do not have the same access to professional knowledge and also over subordinate professionals who are not trained as extensively (professional dominance). This Weberian theory of professional activity allows us to understand some of the finer processes of negotiation on the part of stakeholders which take place in the policy formation process (following Alford and Marmor).

Interest-group work has also been analysed by neo-Marxians such as Habermas (1971). He emphasises that medical knowledge is not value free (or neutral) but that it reflects the cognitive interests of a professional group (doctors) in controlling and predicting disease. This is relevant to the policy-making process in terms of the confidence that other stakeholders have in the legitimacy of psychiatric knowledge.

In psychiatry more than other medical specialities (with the possible exception of obstetrics) there has been a legitimation crisis about the credibility of medical theory and practice. This is evident in the emergence of both 'anti-psychiatry' and a sustained and campaign-focused service-user protest movement (see Chapter 6). It is in the context of this legitimation crisis that mental hospitals became discredited during this century. The work of Goodwin (1997) discussed in Chapter 4 places an emphasis within this neo-Marxian perspective on legitimacy, as well as economic factors, in explaining policy developments.

A contrasting theoretical current, influential recently in sociology, is that of Michel Foucault. His work on the beginnings of psychiatry (Foucault, 1964) was close to a Marxian emphasis on the need for social control. The difference was that whereas Scull emphasised the economic necessity of segregative psychiatry, Foucault emphasised the moral offence created by madness, which led to its rejection by the non-mad in society. Later writers following Foucault suggested that after the segregative and coercive emphasis of early psychiatry, its field of interest broadened to include voluntary relationships in community settings, such as psychological therapies (Castel, Castel and Lovell, 1979; Rose, 1990). This marked a shift from an external form of regulation of the population to one which is based more on self-surveillance.

A final sociological theory which is relevant is that traceable to the work of Durkheim which is more appropriately addressed under the next sub-heading.

Public Health Perspectives and Epidemiology

What is unusual about mental health problems is that although no one has ever claimed or proved that they are transmissible like infectious diseases, they have been treated as if that were the case (Jodelet, 1991). Asylums and sewers were the first two main public health measures imposed by central government in the mid-nineteenth century. This juxtaposition of sewerage and madness might suggest that lunatics were considered to be human waste. This is not such a fanciful notion when the emerging ideology for segregation is uncovered: eugenics. As we will see in the next chapter, late nineteenth-century asylum psychiatry was closely dependent on the underlying assumption that madness was biologically determined. In turn this was part of a wider assumption common in medical scientific (and governmental) culture which held that a variety of deviant states in the lower classes was a function of inferior inheritance.

This core assumption at the turn of this century about the genetic determination of deviance had two opposing consequences in Western psychiatry. On the one hand there were signs, in some countries in the first part of the twentieth century, that the eugenic position went into the ascendant and became more extreme in its policy consequences. The segregation of madness from society, and between the sexes within the asylums to minimise the inheritance of purported faulty genes, had been a convergent policy in Europe and North America. This measure was then amplified to include sterilisation of patients in Denmark and the USA, and extended further in the 1930s in Germany when the German Medical Association proposed a policy of involuntary euthanasia for 'life devoid of meaning'. This meant killing people with learning difficulties, physical disabilities and those diagnosed as being mentally ill. Up to half a million patients in these categories were killed lawfully by German doctors between 1939 and 1942 in health settings. These killings were endorsed by Hitler but not proposed by him.

However, as we will see in Chapters 3 and 4, there was a conflicting consequence of nineteenth-century eugenics, and that was its modification by a new environmentalism. This meant that bio-determinism remained a common assumption in psychiatry but that it was joined by theories which emphasised environmental causes of mental illness.

A common feature of both biological and environmental versions of psychiatric theory is that they accepted that mental illness existed and that it had causes. The opposing theories differed only over the source of these causes. It is here that Durkheim's positivistic view about the reality of social as well as natural phenomena is relevant. It fed into a tradition in social science (traceable to the medical surveys in the eighteenth century) which were directed towards political intervention to prevent ill health (Rosen, 1979; Turner, 1990). Social medicine was in the environmentalist tradition, associated with epidemiology, which was challenged by eugenics and a form of medicine emphasising the pathology within individuals in the late nineteenth century. However, whilst there was a eugenic emphasis in the theoretical developments of psychiatry by 1900, earlier – in the mid-nineteenth century – both physical and psychological ('moral') causes were recorded for lunacy (Hunter and MacAlpine, 1964). Moreover, even though physical causes predominated in records, these were mainly ascribed to environmental rather than genetic events.

By the nineteenth century, decisions about regulating disease levels in the population by government policies were reliant on epidemiological data. The asylums kept detailed records of the conditions of inmates and their ascribed causes. This has had two important consequences for twentieth-century policy formation. First, data collection became an ongoing part of the state bureaucracy. Clinical professionals, hospital administrators and civil servants spent (and still spend) much of their time recording and exchanging information about the prevalence and incidence of psychiatric diagnoses.

A second consequence was the continued legitimacy of a version of social medicine. In the case of psychiatry this meant the emergence of *social psychiatry*, a hybrid discipline of psychiatrists and social scientists. Sometimes medical and social scientists co-operated in large surveys (Hollingshead and Redlich, 1958) or in studying the environmental impact of different hospital regimes (Brown and Wing, 1962). This acceptance of the non-problematic reality of mental illness has entailed some social scientists using epidemiological methods to test theories about its social causation (e.g., Brown and Harris, 1978; Newton, 1988).

Epidemiology can provide data to make decisions about the organisation of psychiatry but it has no conceptual capacity (cf. the other sociological and political science approaches above) to deal with problems of legitimacy in psychiatric theory and practice. It also has nothing to say about stakeholders and the dynamics of their transactions. Its emphasis on measurement means that it offers precise information about the status quo, but it provides no necessary rationale about what to do with that information in the future. Thus it can potentially be used, or co-opted, by all stakeholders involved in policy formation. Its contribution to policy has increased in the last few years where there has been a growing emphasis on 'public health'. Mental health has featured significantly in this regard.

Epidemiological data provides important information on the incidence and prevalence of mental health problems and, by implication, the adequacy or otherwise of existing policies and services to deal with the problem. For example, there is evidence that in the past two decades the suicide rate in young people has risen in the UK (Appleby, *et al.*, 1999). Such evidence might suggest that the policy initiatives aimed at reducing the suicide rates introduced over the same period have not been successful. Thus epidemiology offers a tangible data base in the midst of ignorance and uncertainty in mental health debates. However, a final problem to note about psychiatric epidemiology is that a strong epidemiology includes data on the distribution of causes, and not just diagnoses, in a population. Because the aetiology of functional mental illness remains elusive and contested, psychiatric epidemiology is not able to include causal information and is thus weak. We return to the problems associated with psychiatric epidemiology in Chapter 12.

Comparative Mental Health Policy Analysis

Above, we have assessed some of the strengths and weaknesses of four disciplinary approaches to understanding and interpreting policy formation and development in the mental health field. However, as Goodwin (1997) has pointed out in his analyis of mental health policy in Western Europe and North America, traditional theoretical frameworks have failed to predict policy developments within late capitalist welfare states accurately. Comparative social policy analysis has the added advantage of engaging and learning from the specific experiences of different countries. This can be both historical and contemporary and involve a range of methodologies and sources of data. In general terms, comparative analyses complement more general theories which utilise concepts of structure, agency, economy and polity as explanatory frameworks. Arguments for the utility of comparative policy analysis in the mental health field are provided by Mangen (1994) in discussing his approach to the analysis of the emergence of continuing care practice and policies in European countries. He states that:

> Comparative analysis is an antidote to the generally highly localised implication of results of research of service settings: by testing the equivalent relevance of the concept in a sample of countries, cross-national treatment sharpens the parameters of the problematic, critically refining assessments of generalizability and identifying specificities peculiar to location. The ultimate scientific purpose, of course, is to generate robust explanatory models that hold over space. (Mangen, 1994, 235)

Comparative analysis of systems of cultural beliefs about mental health are also important in understanding prevailing systems of care and adoption of particular policy and practices:

> Cultural belief systems inform whether deviant behaviours are identified and classified as illness, the concepts of etiology and cure, and the designation of appropriate healers. In any cultural system, modal concepts of mental illness, help-seeking paths, and utilisation patterns are intermeshed with the organisation and structure of service delivery systems . . . Additionally, a culture's assessed needs for social control and order, its prevailing philosophies and legal protections, and its economic organization and resources all have had a significant impact on the structure of mental health service delivery systems. (Lefley 1999, 567)

Comparative analysis draws attention to global similarities and the identification of broad general developments. Goodwin (1997) highlights the common patterns and trends in mental health systems across a variety of countries in the second part of the twentieth century. He points to the establishment of a variety of insurance-based schemes alongside fewer countries adopting services funded from general taxation; a trend away from reliance upon long-term hospitalisation towards an eclectic and variegated community-based system of services and management; and a reduction in the availability of institutionalised care.

There are also cross-national differences, as well as similarities, which are pointed up by making comparisons between different countries. Whilst there is a global convergence in the existence of compulsory powers of detention and a world wide trend towards the medicalisation of madness, there are differences in compulsory detention legislation across different countries. This variability reflects a variable relationship between the State, civil society and the use of mental health powers. Each state in the USA passes its own mental health legislation resulting in a diversity of commitment systems and the heterogeneous application of therapeutic law. Over the past ten years Japan has incarcerated many more patients on an involuntary basis than European countries. Perhaps this reflects the gravity with which transgressions of social norms are viewed in Japanese society. By contrast, in Italy compulsory admission procedures are partly a civil matter signified by the involvement of the mayor in compulsory admission proceedings. This may be linked to the Italian tradition of participatory involvement of people in civil, legal and health provision.

Comparative analyses over time within countries is also illuminating. Currently in the UK, the focus on public safety and a downplaying of civil libertarian values (a hallmark of the social polices of 'New Labour') have been accompanied by an emphasis on new compulsory powers 'to convey to hospital' in the event of non-compliance with treatment in the community. Such powers had previously been considered but rejected on pragmatic as well as civil libertarian grounds by a Conservative administration (see Chapter 12).

Conclusion

This first chapter has introduced some arguments about the utility of different approaches to policy formation. A salient point is that policy formation (about mental health or anything else) can be fruitfully understood using an inter-disciplinary framework, which spans the whole of social science and extends, in our case, into social medicine. We emphasise this point elsewhere when discussing the need to understand mental health policy broadly at three levels: macro, meso and micro (Pilgrim and Rogers, 1999). The first of these refers to global and trans-historical trends, the second to current national social administrative arrangements and the third to the social-psychological processes in the development of retention of policy in localities and by individuals and groups. Our process emphasis in the book was highlighted in the preface but we recognise that some students of social policy may wish to focus on the social administrative detail of current or past British mental health legislation. As far as current policy is concerned, this is outlined in the middle of Chapter 12. We will also outline some relevant historical features in Chapters 3 and 4. Before that, in the next chapter, we examine the different perspectives of the various interest groups associated with mental health policy debates.

2

Interest Groups and their Perspectives

Introduction

The mental health care policy arena, like other areas of health and social care, involves a number of social groups which at times hold different sets of interests. They also subscribe to varying perspectives of mental health. A 'medicalised' view of 'mental illness' dominates mental health policy and practice both in the UK and in most other countries. However, there is none the less a diversity of conceptualisations of mental health and illness which influence the making and development of mental health policy and the nature of practice.

The debate about whether we should use competing terms such as 'madness', 'mental illness', 'mental distress', 'mental health problems', 'freaking out' and 'mental disorder' is not only about semantic disagreements: these terms are products of different interest groups. For example, 'mental disorder' is essentially a legal category, whereas 'mental illness' is a medical one. For now we will clarify why they are different and to what degree they are compatible. Thus this second chapter will introduce two issues: the range of interest groups involved in mental health debates; and the different ways in which mental health has been conceptualised and viewed within contemporary society. In other words, *who* are the people constituting interest groups and *how* do they view mental health?

Interest Groups and Mental Health Policy

Williamson (1993) provides a definition of interests and 'stakes' which can usefully be applied to the personnel operating within the structure and organisation of mental health provision:

19

Interests are to do with advantage and detriment to individuals and to groups. Interests . . . are something in which a stake is held; a personal or group resource or means to protect or enhance a resource. Everyone has interests in resources like influence, power, time, money, knowledge, the way situations involving themselves are defined. (Williamson, 1993, 3)

Different groups have different degrees of power and influence. The latter are not static but change over time and according to the issue. Some groups have a defined occupational interest in framing mental health problems in certain ways. These 'dominant' interests tend to predominate over those of other stakeholders. For their part the other groups are not disinterested. They are less preoccupied with occupational status and salaries except as a possible target of criticism and more concerned about the sources of their own mental disability or the offence, burden or disruption caused by others. Some, such as the police and those working in the criminal justice system, also have to deal with mental health problems and so have a perspective to be noted. This is true also of the managers and commissioners of services. These have considerable influence over mental health service provision but lack a distinct coherent disciplinary notion of mental health. Let us look at these interest groups and their perspectives in a little more detail.

The Mental Health Specialists

The occupational groups which claim an expertise in mental health, sometimes called the 'psy complex', include psychiatrists, clinical psychologists, psychiatric social workers, psychiatric nurses, psychoanalysts, psychotherapists and counsellors. In Chapter 5 we will go into more detail about the relationship between the state and the different mental health occupations. Here the perspectives held by different expert groups will be noted.

Psychiatrists

Psychiatrists are trained in medicine and so they tend to emphasise diagnosis, treatment, prognosis (predicting the outcome of an illness) and aetiology (speculating about its cause). In the latter regard, the bodily emphasis of medical training and its social history ensure that biological/chemical or physiological causes have been privileged. This has led, in the main, to treatment approaches dominated by drugs and other somatic interventions. In the nineteenth century biological theories of madness prevailed and this has left a strong impact on psychiatric thinking even a century later (see Chapter 3). In the twentieth century, psychiatrists have become more eclectic in their aetiological theories. Many of them now accept social and psychological causes of mental illness, as well as biological ones. They also use psychological as well as somatic treatments, although the latter still predominate. The new eclectic psychiatry emphasises all three sources of causation in its 'biopsychosocial' model (see, e.g., Falloon and Fadden, 1993). The traditionally dominant role of psychiatrists in services is reflected in the terms 'psychiatric hospital' and 'psychiatric nurses' and 'psychiatric social workers'. Indeed, until recently the term 'psychiatry' had become a catch-all phrase to include not just a medical specialty but its associated facilities and subordinated occupational groups. More recently, Community Psychiatric Nurses have dropped the term 'psychiatric' for the preferred 'Community Mental Health Nurse', signalling perhaps a dilution of the impact of medical authority.

Clinical psychologists

Clinical psychologists are a relatively new group. Their occupation was officially recognised by the title of 'clinical psychologist' with the introduction of the NHS (Dabbs, 1972). They hold a variety of theoretical positions, which reflect competing models in their academic discipline. Thus psychoanalysis, behaviourism, humanistic psychology and cognitivism are all represented in the work of clinical psychology practitioners (Goldie, 1974; Pilgrim and Treacher, 1992). These are divergent and often antagonistic models of human functioning. Consequently, 'psychologically-orientated' mental health work has no coherent and agreed way of theorising about the problems of service recipients.

Psychoanalysis and other forms of depth psychology emphasise the role of the unconscious mind. By contrast, behaviourism only considers external aspects of conduct to be amenable to scientific description and systematic and measurable modification. Humanistic psychology emphasises subjectivity and the potential of human beings to grow, given the correct personal circumstances. Like psychoanalysis, this implies the provision of some form of psychotherapy. Cognitivism emphasises the role of thought processes in human functioning. Whereas behavioural treatments (such as the use of 'token economies') emphasise

changing outer behaviour, cognitive therapies emphasise the modification of thought processes. Despite this plethora of apparently contradictory
theoretical positions, clinical psychologists have developed an array of
hybrid and eclectic mixtures for themselves in their assessment techniques and therapeutic practice.

Unlike GPs, psychiatrists, nurses, social workers and police officers,
psychologists hold no legal powers of detention under mental health
legislation. For this reason, in comparison with the other mental health
occupations, the influence which they exert flows more from their theoretical knowledge and therapeutic credibility than from their organisational
power or position.

Psychiatric nurses

Compared with psychiatry and psychology, the knowledge base of nursing
is less well developed. As in other branches of nursing, psychiatric
nurses have traditionally been subordinate to medicine. Consequently,
they have not developed a separate body of knowledge. In practice
they follow the contours of more academically-based disciplines (psychiatry, clinical psychology and sociology). More recent changes in
the curriculum of psychiatric nurse training suggest that reactions against
medical theory (embracing more social and psychological models) have
been associated with attempts to shift towards greater professional
autonomy. The practice of psychiatric nurses is discussed in detail in
Chapter 5.

Social workers

Social workers who are specially trained to fulfil their duties under the
1983 Mental Health Act are more likely to import a social perspective
into mental health work. In part this stems from their different occupational roots. Psychiatrists, clinical psychologists and psychiatric nurses
arose within, or as a result of, the asylum system. The modern occupational location of social work is different. Its recent development is
embedded in local authority social service structures with a focus on
'community' working and links. However, this does not necessarily
imply a coherent theoretical approach to social work. Social science
itself is internally divided about the topic of mental abnormality. Two
broad strands of sociological thought can be identified as having influenced social work training and practice in mental health. First, a social
causation approach accepts the existence of mental illness but seeks to

identify its social determinants (e.g., the stresses of poverty or racial or sexual disadvantage). Second, social reaction or labelling theory emphasises the role of the reactions of others to deviance in its maintenance and amplification (Scheff, 1966). Whilst a social focus is often referred to in social work theory and training, in practice social workers often follow a medical model of mental illness in their everyday work (Goldie, 1974; Bean, 1979). Psychoanalytic ideas have also been influential in case work both inside and outside mental health work.

Psychoanalysts

Psychoanalysts are drawn from a number of occupational groups but psychiatrists tend to dominate their training institutes. (Non-medical practitioners are still called 'lay analysts'.) Psychoanalysis was invented by Sigmund Freud but his modern-day followers are divided into those following his ideas, those of Melanie Klein, and others who draw eclectically from these two main sources. Freud focused on explaining the unconscious basis of neurotic symptoms and later analysts examined the early infantile sources of depression (Bowlby, 1969) and psychosis (Winnicott, 1958; Laing, 1967). This spread of interest within psychoanalysts reflects theoretical splits about both the age at which mental health problems are assumed to begin and also the role of the instincts versus quality of parenting.

Psychoanalysts conceptualise mental health problems in terms of a hierarchy of fixation at, or regression to, earlier forms of psychological functioning in a person's life. Neurotic anxiety, for instance, might be seen as an outcome of unresolved sexual feelings about a parent. Depression might be understood as resulting from early difficulties around separation from a parent. Psychosis could be understood as a failure to be nurtured and made secure in the very earliest months of a person's life. Over the last 50 years psychoanalysis as a body of knowledge has had considerable influence on social, as well as mental health, policy and practice. This has been seen as having both a positive and negative effect. Comments by two of the leading social policy analysts, Richard Titmuss and Barbara Wootton (writing in the 1950s), illustrate the point. Titmuss writes of psychoanalysis in almost messianic terms:

> the work of Freud and his successors has been of revolutionary importance to medicine; it has changed our attitudes to the mentally ill, it has at least helped towards the alleviation of mental suffering,

it has enlarged the possibilities of preventative therapy, and it has given us new ways of looking at the growth of personality and the origins of illness ... it has for, doctors and laymen alike, undermined our psychological innocence, sensitised us to an inner world of reality, and made us see all sickness, in whatever guise, as part of a psychological continuum (Titmuss, 1958, 107)

By contrast, Wootton expresses dismay and contempt at the end of a discussion about the pervasiveness of psychoanalytical ideas in social work texts, which she views as a trend which disguises the social and economic root of people's problems:

Happily, it can be presumed that the lamentable arrogance of the [psychoanalytical] language in which contemporary social workers describe their activities is not generally matched by the work that they actually do: otherwise it is hardly credible that they would not constantly get their faces slapped. Happily, also, the literature of social work is not generally read by those who receive its administrations. Without doubt the majority of those who engage in social work are sensible, practical people who conduct their business in a reasonably matter-of-fact basis. The pity is that they have to write such nonsense about it: and to present themselves to the world as so deeply tainted with what Virginia Woolf has called 'the peculiar repulsiveness of those who dabble their fingers self approvingly in the stuff of others' souls'. (Wootton, 1959, 279)

Psychotherapists and counsellors also work in statutory and voluntary educational and health settings. Their theoretical approaches may be drawn from psychoanalysis, behaviourism, cognitivism or humanistic psychology. This last category (for instance, following the work of Carl Rogers) has been particularly influential in voluntary sector mental health services such as The Samaritans and Marriage Guidance (now Relate).

Non-specialists

The 'paraprofessionals'

De Swaan (1990) has pointed out that a layer of professionals exists outside the psy complex, including GPs, the clergy, teachers, probation officers and the police, who make decisions about mental health problems and may play a temporary or partial role in actually working with psychiatric patients. From what we know about this group, they seem to form a bridge between mental health experts and patients and the general public. They generally have a role in detecting mental health problems and making decisions about whether to get more formal psychiatric agencies involved. They also provide a role in support through talking and advice, and perhaps mobilising lay and community resources that lie outside the domain of formal services.

Paraprofessionals use a mixture of ordinary and expert under-standings. For instance, a study of the understanding that the police have about mental health problems when operating Section 136 of the Mental Health Act suggests that they use commonsense judgements about people they consider to have a mental health problem found in public places (Rogers, 1990).

Politicians and civil servants

The legal and medical perspectives are endorsed by parliamentary politicians and subsequently by civil servants serving government. They also provide a framework of duty and constraint for mental health service managers. Politicians creating and changing legislation have wider powers of influence over mental health than mental health legislation. Additionally, they are responsible for other legislation (for instance, about health care organisation, employment, housing and income maintenance) which impinges on mental health service-users. In the 1990s, the 1983 Mental Health Act probably had less of an influence on service development than a different piece of legislation, the 1990 NHS and Community Care Act.

The views of governing politicians about mental health and mental health policy-making have been researched little. However, Ramon (1985) documents the views of politicians about mental health legislation in the 1920s and 1950s. A number of features were present which are likely to be relevant considerations still today.

1 Mental health is not a high priority for most MPs.
2 Views about the topic do not always fall neatly into party political perspectives. In relation to civil liberties, there is frequently a shared libertarian concern in debates which cross party lines.
3 MPs and government ministers are sensitive to public opinion and prejudice. Whether this is about the wrongful detention of the sane or fears about dangerous patients in the community, it is clear that

mental health policy may often be shaped by the proxy interests of a voting public, as interpreted by politicians. People with mental health problems are themselves a minority voting group. This is a relatively new phenomenon. Patients in psychiatric hospitals did not have the vote prior to the 1983 Mental Health Act.

4   A minority of parliamentarians may become product champions' for mental health policy often because of their own personal experience or interests. Examples here are the Conservative Donald MacIntosh in the 1950s who was not only a doctor but also an ex-mental patient. In 1992 Ian McCartney, as an opposition Labour MP, was instrumental in setting up a policy review of mental health as a priority area of health policy by the Parliamentary Labour Party. Tessa Jowell, another Labour MP and ex-training and education director for MIND, has also sponsored a private member's bill in response to government proposals for supervised discharge orders. The former Secretary of State for Health, Virginia Bottomley, was an ex-psychiatric social worker and this was a relevant influential factor in past debates about mental health policy and services.

Below politicians are groups of civil servants who also may define or shape policy in their advice to ministers. A sub-group of these will be indirectly representing professional interests as they are appointed as medical or nursing officers in the Department of Health or as mental health leads in the Regional NHS Executive. The influence of civil servants on ministerial decision-making varies. Recently the traditional function of the advisory role between civil servants and politicians may have been weakened by ministers seeking information and advice from other sources. For example, the Internal Reference Group (IRG) set up in 1997 was constituted by a disparate range of representatives from professional, voluntary and other organisations concerned with mental health. This effectively by-passed the traditional role of civil servants in collecting evidence and advising ministers on the most appropriate course of action to take.

Collectively, too, the role played by central government agencies and agents in implementing directives and programmes varies. For example, during the 1990s a more directive role was taken by civil servants and ministers working from within central government agencies. This replaced the previous oscillation between prescription and a more *laissez-faire* approach to service developments where the emphasis was on local enthusiasm (or absence of it) for initiatives. The Department of Health advocated the need for mental health services to foster partnerships between health, local authorities and GP fundholders and closer working between providers, carers and users of services (DH, 1995). Mechanisms for ensuring this were linked to obtaining resources for services (e.g., via the Mental Illness Specific Grant scheme). Civil servants based in the Regional Offices of the NHS Executive (NHSE) undertook visits with members of the Social Services Inspectorate to monitor the progress of mental health service commissioning. It is likely that the experience gained from these centralised initiatives subsequently influenced the development of policy-making about partnerships and a 'joined up' approach to services emphasising the relevance of a social care agenda.

Service managers

A range of managers responsible for commissioning and providing mental health services exists in each locality. These have a variety of personal and professional experiences of mental health services and are located across a variety of settings, such as local authorities, primary care groups and NHS Trusts. They are constrained by central government policy but can also exercise considerable discretion about engendering or retarding local policy initiatives. Commissioning managers have had a significant role to play in setting and monitoring the performance of provider units by their specifications in contracts. This contractual control allows the importation of expectations about service type in a locality. There is an increasing trend for these to be based on 'evidence' and guidelines regarding good practice, but a preference for what is included is also likely to be influenced by the personal values and attitudes of managers towards mental health. They may also exercise discretion over the types of service which are bought within their allocated budget.

Commissioners of services also represent an important countervailing power to that of local clinical interests within the NHS (though at times they represent both). As well as having their own pre-existing views about what should constitute a good local mental health service, they are open to local lobbies, such as advocacy and self-advocacy groups. Recently managers have also become more powerful in the generation of patterns of services and mental health practice in a locality, particularly with regard to community services. Community mental health centres and teams were originally initially locality-led by 'product champions'. These were either consultant psychiatrists influenced by developments in the USA or inter-disciplinary teams who wished to set up alternatives to the limited range of psychiatric services in a locality. Managerial arrangements tended to follow the existing structures and professional arrangements. Later the proliferation of community mental health teams (CMHTs), which became part of national policy (DH, 1995), came to depend more on managerial action in ensuring the implementation of the necessary components of local mental health services.

During the 1990s, the complexity of professional versus managerial authority and arrangements in managing CMHTs were problematic (Onyett, Standen and Peck 1997). Until the late 1990s there had been a fairly clear demarcation between 'purchasers' and 'providers'. The 1980s had seen a general trend towards a greater role for managers. The internal market arrangements which were introduced in 1991 extended the influence of managers further in both their purchasing and providing authority. It is likely that with the abolition of the internal market, with its culture of competition, that managers as a formal group will hold less sway over the shape of services than will the multi-disciplinary clinical groupings being created by the newer arrangements of 'clinical governance' (see Chapters 5 and 12).

Differing Views about Mental Health

Given the wide divergence of theoretical perspectives within the occupational groups described earlier, it is clear that collectively they share no common theory of mind and behaviour. It is not as if there is a broad consensus which contains conflicts of opinion. Instead, theoretical polarisations can be identified about a number of issues. In particular, splits occur between:

(a) those emphasising biological or inherited tendencies towards mental abnormality versus those emphasising environmental factors;
(b) those emphasising internal events (thoughts and feelings) and those emphasising behaviour;
(c) those emphasising causes and those emphasising consequences of mental abnormality;
(d) those emphasising an eclectic inclusion of biological, psychological and social factors versus those privileging one group of these factors.

A practical consequence of this mixture of ideas is that service recipients encounter a wider range of interventions, which sit more or less easily together. For example, in relation to rehabilitation, Bean and Mounser (1993) describe a typical treatment approach thus: 'A man being resettled after developing schizophrenia may receive medication (medical model) in a hostel run on therapeutic community lines (social model) whilst receiving social skills training (behavioural model)' (Bean and Mounser, 1993, 31).

The knowledge produced and used by professionals is not composed of static entities divorced from policy formation processes; rather, professional ideas about the nature and treatment of mental health problems impact on policy formation which in turn feeds back into professional knowledge. For example, the differentiation of services for different groups in the nineteenth century is related to different notions about emotional and intellectual deviance. Prior to the 1890 Lunacy Act an elaborate network of asylums had been built (see Chapter 3) which contained 'aments', now known as people with learning difficulties or disabilities, as well as 'demerits' or 'lunatics'. As 'mental illness' and 'mental handicap' came to be seen as separate specialisms with distinct bodies of knowledge, so these were distinguished from one another in policy legislation and provision. The advent of community care policies has also heralded changes in the conceptualisation of disease categories within psychiatry, which have made the task of detecting and managing madness in non-institutional settings by psychiatry easier. We expand on this point in Chapter 5.

The legal perspective

Another example of theorising mental abnormality can be found in mental health legislation. The 1983 Mental Health Act, passed by politicians and drawn up by lawyers, has an explicit account of mental abnormality. However, in legal terms 'mental disorder' refers to more than 'mental illness'. The Act includes four types of mental disorder:

(a) mental illness – this is not defined;
(b) mental impairment – this refers to people with learning difficulties who are also deemed to be abnormally aggressive;
(c) severe mental impairment – this refers to people with severe learning difficulties who are also deemed to be abnormally aggressive;
(d) psychopathic disorder – this refers to anti-social individuals who are 'abnormally aggressive' or who manifest 'seriously irresponsible conduct'.

Thus, the legal perspective offers four explicit categorisations of mental abnormality but offers little beyond that given by psychiatric experts. Mental illness is not defined, so its existence in law must remain parasitic on the views given by psychiatrists. Similarly, the third and fourth categories rely on an expert (psychiatric or clinical psychological) view about learning difficulty combined with a judgement about dangerousness. The final category is completely circular and so has little explanatory value. People are judged to be psychopathic because of their dangerous and anti-social acts, and they are deemed to be dangerous and anti-social because they are suffering from a psychopathic disorder. This would seem to offer little improvement on the explanatory power of the notion of 'evil'.

Whatever the theoretical weaknesses of a legal view about mental abnormality, it has great practical significance. As we will see in later chapters, the courts have been involved in admitting people to psychiatric facilities over a long period. Since 1959 those powers have been substantially reduced, but even today the courts are still involved where judgements are made about mentally disordered offenders. Also, lawyers are involved on Mental Health Review Tribunals, when decisions are made about the discharge of both offender and non-offender patients held under varying sections of the Mental Health Act.

The lay perspective

The gap created by the absence of a legal definition of mental illness has led to variable outcomes in court decision-making and rulings about mental disorder in society. For instance, expert witnesses for both the defence and prosecution examining Peter Sutcliffe ('The Yorkshire Ripper') agreed that he was suffering from paranoid schizophrenia when he murdered a series of women. However, the jury of lay people found him guilty of malice aforethought and he was sent to prison, not a secure hospital. (After the judgement he was transferred from prison to a Special Hospital.) In the case of Dennis Nilson who killed, dismembered and stored fifteen young men in his flat, the defence expert witness argued he suffered from a psychopathic disorder but the one for the prosecution did not. He was also sent to prison.

These examples demonstrate that lay people are in a position to overrule expert judgements about mental disorder. Moreover, as an indication of the difficulty the criminal justice system has in making distinctions between mental normality and abnormality, here is an example of an opinion given by Judge Lawton in 1974. He said that the words 'mental illness' are 'ordinary words of the English language. They have no particular medical significance. They have no particular legal significance.' Lawton refers back to a ruling given by Law Lord Reid, who was talking of an offender whose sanity was in doubt: 'I ask myself what would the ordinary sensible person have said about the patient's condition in this case if he [*sic*] had been informed of his behaviour? In my judgment such a person would have said "Well the fellow is obviously mentally ill."' (Cited in R. Jones, 1991, p. 15.)

Hoggett (1990) points out that this has been called 'the man(*sic*)-must-be-mad' test. In other words, in order to carry out act *X*, the person must have been crazy. This highlights what is at the heart of lay judgements about madness: the unintelligibility of acts. What Lawton may have been trying to express by his use of the word 'significance' was really 'validity' or even 'utility', when the term 'mental illness' is used. In other words, the term 'mental illness' does not get us very far beyond the situation that when a person's conduct in its context cannot be understood, this leads to a judgement that the action is 'mad'. A diagnosis of mental illness merely puts a technical gloss on this lay judgement.

This suggests that ordinary conceptions of madness or unintelligible conduct may approximate to psychiatric diagnoses of psychosis. Coulter (1973), in his study of everyday judgements about madness, pointed out that lay people are involved in making decisions about mental illness which are then rubber-stamped as formal diagnoses by professionals called in to deal with crises. As evidence of the proximity of the lay discourse to judgements made by psychiatrists, the study on psychiatric referrals from the police referred to earlier showed that the police were as reliable in their judgements as experts about the presence or absence of mental illness, which was confirmed by psychiatric diagnosis after a police referral. However, experts and non-experts making judgements about mental abnormality may not always concur.

There are two cautions against conflating lay judgements about madness and psychiatric diagnoses. First, as we have already noted in the cases of Sutcliffe and Nilson, lay people may believe someone to be sane when psychiatrists believe them to be suffering from mental illness (or psychopathy). Also at times the reverse may apply: Bean (1979) found that psychiatrists sometimes will disagree with relatives who insist that a person is mentally ill. Second, lay people seem to hold a much narrower view about what constitutes mental illness than do psychiatrists. Studies of stereotypes about mental illness (Jones and Cochrane, 1981) show that lay people mainly focus on florid psychotic symptoms, bizarre behaviour, delusions and hallucinations, but ignore the commonest of all psychiatric conditions: depression. The association between violence and mental illness made by lay people is well known. This is both reflected in and reinforced by journalistic accounts of mental illness. In Philo and colleagues' (1996) study about media constructs of mental illness, they found that most items dealing with mental health issues forged a link between mental illness and violence. Respondents with personal knowledge of mental illness accepted the dominant media messages, despite the evidence of their own direct experience of mental health. The exaggerated link between violence and mental health is also discernible in government action and policy statements, and is an association that is pointed up during political debates about the availability of services, indicating the sensitivity of mental health policy-makers to this public concern.

Lay people may hold different views according to their circumstances. The parents of a disruptive adolescent with a diagnosis of schizophrenia may seek a response from mental health practitioners that differs from the response sought by the identified patient. This is shown up at the collective level by the conflicting demands about services made by organised interest groups. Groups which have tended to see themselves as mainly representing relatives' interests (such as SANE, or Schizophrenia A National Emergency) have tended to focus on the need for hospital beds and for interventions to be imposed more frequently against resistant patients. The reverse can then be found in the demands of service-user groups such as Survivors Speak Out. They want less coercion, fewer inpatient facilities and more social support and help in ordinary environments. The recent trend of consumerism in health care has increased the credence of such views (see Chapter 6). Also, if lay people are asked to explore the notion of mental health, they can elaborate their own version of 'lay epidemiology' (Rogers and Pilgrim, 1997) indicating that superficial stereotyping and richer accounts can co-exist.

Identifying and measuring those with mental health problems

The diversity of opinion about the causes and nature of mental health problems amongst the different interest groups means that it is not an easy matter to specify which people in society constitute those with a mental health problem. A definition based on service contact only captures the group of people with mental health problems who enter the role of patient. In this regard, mental health and physical health are similar. Community surveys point up a 'clinical iceberg' (Hannay, 1979) with many more people experiencing symptoms than are diagnosed by professionals. For example, Goldberg and Huxley (1992) suggest the prevalence levels shown in Table 2.1.

TABLE 2.1 *Five levels and four filters, with estimates of annual point prevalence rates at each level*

Level 1 The community
                260–315/1000/year
.... 1st filter
                                                                        (Illness behaviour)
Level 2 Total mental morbidity – attenders in primary care
                230/1000/year
....2nd filter
                                                                    (Ability to detect disorder)
Level 3 Mental disorders identified by doctors ('Conspicuous Psychiatric
             Morbidity')
                101.5/1000/year
.... 3rd filter
                                                        (Referral to mental illness services)
Level 4 Total morbidity – mental illness services
                23.5/1000/year
....4th filter
                                                            (Admission to psychiatric beds)
Level 5 Psychiatric inpatients
                5.71/1000/year

Source: adapted from Goldberg and Huxley (1992).

This model of prevalence attempts to use diagnosed and undiagnosed groups in society to define those with mental health problems. Those objecting to psychiatric diagnosis on moral or scientific grounds may be uneasy with this formulation (see Chapter 11). None the less, it is a starting point to think about the scale of mental distress and oddity in society. Unfortunately, even those committed to a medical diagnostic or epidemiological framework offer no certain consensus about prevalence. Prevalence refers to the number of people with a particular illness at a point in time in a population. Incidence refers to new cases. Within a psychiatric epidemiological framework, results of prevalence studies differ greatly. For example, in relation to 'schizophrenia', estimates vary from rates of 1:2000 to 1:100 adults. Variations are due to differences in diagnostic practices of psychiatrists, but also to social and environmental factors (Warner, 1985). More recently, psychiatric epidemiology has used symptom-based measures rather than relying on simplistic diagnostic categories to assess the levels of mental health problems in populations. Results from surveys sponsored by the Department of Health carried out in the 1990s (Office of Population and Census Statistics, 1994) provides a picture of the prevalence of mental health problems of adults aged between 16 and 64 living in British households. The main findings are as set out below.

1 The prevalence of neurotic disorders is estimated at 156 per thousand. Women were far more likely to experience neurotic symptoms, and younger women were more likely to experience depression and anxiety than older women. The most common neurotic symptoms were fatigue, sleep problems, irritability and worry.

2 Psychotic disorders are estimated to affect four people in every thousand. Alcohol problem prevalence was estimated at 47 per thousand and drug dependency as 22 per thousand. Men are three times as likely to experience such problems as women, and they are most prevalent amongst young men.

As well as the question of how frequently mental health problems occur being a basis for defining a population, we can also consider other social indicators. For example, whilst all mental health problems, whether defined by diagnosis or by lay accounts of distress and oddity, occur across society, the spread is not random and neither is it even. Prevalence is associated with marital status, rural/urban location, class, sex, age and race. We have examined this point in relation to age, sex, race and class in some depth elsewhere (Pilgrim and Rogers, 1999). Here we summarise some relevant points and give a few examples.

Age About 5 per cent of the child and adolescent population are deemed, by standard psychiatric criteria, to be suffering from conduct or emotional problems (Harrington, 1993). The probability of being newly diagnosed as schizophrenic is relatively high in young adulthood but very low in childhood and old age. Organic changes to the brain increase the probability of a diagnosis of dementia with increasing age. Predictions are that the numbers of those suffering from dementia will increase dramatically in the future. The number of people over 75 years old has increased in the general population by 30 per cent since 1976. Age is also relevant in relation to the correlation between sexual abuse in childhood and the raised probability of mental health problems in later years.

Gender   Women receive a psychiatric diagnosis more frequently than men. The bulk of this difference is accounted for by the higher rates of diagnosis in women of depression. Men receive a diagnosis of personality disorder and commit suicide more often than women and are overrepresented in secure psychiatric facilities.

Race   African Caribbean people in Britain are disproportionately diagnosed as suffering from schizophrenia. Irish people are overrepresented in all diagnostic groups (see Chapter 7).

Class   People with a diagnosis of schizophrenia are disproportionately likely to be poor, although the relationship between cause and effect here is still contested. Some argue that becoming mentally ill creates downward drift in society. Others emphasise that the stress of poverty increases the probability of morbidity.

If we take these variables together, they point to a direct correlation between mental health problems and social disadvantage. As with the note about the clinical iceberg, this correlation is also true of physical health problems. The interaction of the variables can also be noted. The mental health of rich people tends actually to improve in old age, whereas the opposite is true of poor people (Blaxter, 1990). Women live longer than men, on average, and so have a higher probability of suffering from senile dementia. At least some of the raised levels of severe psychiatric morbidity in black people could be attributed to the combined stress of racism and poverty. However, this claim applies more to African Caribbean people than to Asian people in Britain.

Despite these complex interactions and difficulties in tracing cause and effect, it is possible to draw three conclusions about mental health problems and disadvantage. First, people who are already disadvantaged or oppressed have a greater probability of having to contend with the extra burden of mental health problems: the experience of distress and the loss of social credibility associated with a loss of reason. When and if they enter the role of psychiatric patient, they will import all the vulnerabilities of their race, class and gender background. These multiple sources of disadvantage may account for why psychiatric patients have been treated so oppressively within services.

Second, people with mental health problems are more likely to have to contend with additional sources of disadvantage, such as racism, sexism and unemployment, when they attempt to live independently of specialist services. These compound the process of social exclusion resulting directly from the stigma associated with psychiatric diagnosis ('mentalism'). Thus psychiatric patients suffer disadvantage both inside and outside the services they receive. The protection of class privilege may mitigate, but not eliminate, this double disadvantage (for instance, by having a choice of paid therapists and by being able to be unemployed without being poor).

Third, at times the way in which psychiatry and psychiatric researchers have conceptualised the relationship between disadvantage and mental health has militated against an analysis of mental health problems and policy initiatives which tackles the causes and effects of such disadvantage. There has, for example, been a long-standing interest in the relationship between *homelessness and mental health.* Traditionally social scientists have placed the root of the problem of homelessness in the context of poverty, economic disadvantage and social upheaval. From his experiences of being 'down and out' George Orwell vividly depicted the effects on mental health in describing homeless people as those 'who have fallen into solitary half-mad grooves of life and given up trying to be normal or decent. Poverty frees them from ordinary standards of behaviour, just as money frees people from work' (Orwell, 1986). Yet rarely has traditional psychiatric research put poverty centre-stage in examining mental health and homelessness or seen mental distress as a response to homelessness. Rather, a lack of a home has frequently been viewed as the by-product of the personality defects of individuals (Whiteley, 1955). Whilst on the face of things this appears to be an 'interest free' area of research, albeit one that pathologises individuals, some commentators have suggested that professional interests are important in understanding the construction of mental illness and homelessness as a psychiatric problem.

Snow *et al.* (1986) undertook ethnographic fieldwork to assess the mental health status of homeless people in the United States. They found that only 15 per cent of the 911 homeless people the researchers had contact with could be considered as 'mentally ill' (based on criteria of prior institutionalisation, peer identification and observed bizarre and inappropriate behaviour). The authors of the study consider the high prevalence rates previously recorded as in part due to a desire to medicalise problems. Certainly, in Britain, a catastrophic discourse about homelessness and mental health problems accompanied discussions about community care which at the time appeared little more than a thinly veiled attempt to promote the advantages of the Victorian asylums by vested psychiatric interests with not so much as a passing wave to the social disadvantage and needs of homeless people themselves. The latter is much more a concern with wider questions about citizenship than it is to do with the presence or absence of mental pathology.

Conclusion

This second chapter has introduced a variety of interests in the field of mental health. Competing stakeholder perspectives are more common here than elsewhere. For example, whilst medical knowledge in general is contested by academic sociologists, only a few specific areas of medical practice have evoked a passionate and articulate lay critique, one such area being women's health (particularly about obstetric care), and the other mental health. These share particular common features about power and control over the body and the self, and sensitivities about privacy and individuality. Politicians are particularly sensitive about their reading of public fears about mental abnormality. Whereas the public's view on the general state of funding and viability of the NHS has been a focus of political concern in recent years, few specific topics have been debated with as much passion and prejudice as mental health.

Part II

Historical Considerations

3

The Dominance of the Victorian Asylum

Introduction

This chapter, the first of two with a historical emphasis, summarises the factors which led to the emergence of the large asylum system in the nineteenth century. It then outlines the enduring impact this system had on developments up to and including the twentieth century. The next chapter will continue the account, continuing the story from the Second World War to the present.

The English 'Great Confinement'?

Foucault (1961) maintained that from the mid-seventeenth century a 'great confinement' took place across Europe. However, the course of English developments did not follow this depiction. During this period, by and large, *non-institutionalised*, privatised means of dealing with all deviant groups prevailed. From 1660 onwards social life was still characterised by parochialism. Throughout the Middle Ages and beyond there was an absence of formal provision. It was not until after 1780, when the numbers of madhouses grew rapidly, that an era dedicated to the confinement of lunacy began in England. There were 16 metropolitan licensed houses in 1774, but by 1819 there were 40.

The last quarter of the eighteenth century and first quarter of the nineteenth century saw a dramatic move away from unregulated, *ad hoc* local arrangements to a system which was increasingly segregative, centralised and managed. Madhouses were not seen as panaceas; even then there was a public distaste for confining people. They remained diverse and small scale and were typical of eighteenth-century institutions in being characterised by heterogeneity. The establishment of public asylums changed all of this, replacing it with a panoptic rational centralised system of discipline specifically aimed at catering for the lunatic.

By the end of the eighteenth century, a number of institutions following the path of the growth of the voluntary hospital movement had emerged. Funded out of public donations, these have been viewed by Porter (1987) as the first wave of public asylums. These institutions had a broader-based clientele than the madhouses and were generally set up to cater for respectable local citizens and the 'deserving' poorer classes. Smaller establishments included the ward for incurable lunatics at Guy's Hospital, established in 1728. St Luke's Hospital, which opened in London in 1751, was a larger enterprise, as was a lunatic hospital established in Manchester in 1766. Similar organisations sprang up in other major cities in the second half of the century (York, Liverpool, Leicester and Exeter).

Insanity: a medical or moral issue?

Charitably-funded facilities were often part of a hospital, attached to infirmaries or named 'lunatic hospitals'. Some were founded by eminent mad-doctors wishing to promote their medical sub-specialty. According to Scull (1979, 25), St Luke's 'represented a major attempt to assert medical control over the problem of insanity'. It banned casual sightseeing, the hallmark of Bedlam, incorporated 'asylum' (with its connotation of 'sanctuary') into its title, and indicated its commitment to medical science by accommodating medical students.

The development and acceptance of a medical model of insanity was characterised by a number of features. There was the construction of a theory, which defined madness as a medical category with a biological basis. The beginning of the nineteenth century saw a proliferation of medical categories with specified symptoms and aetiology. The causes of medical insanity were conceived to be inside the person; they were a result of physical imbalances and an eruption of nature. Masturbation and its consequent spermatorrhoea (excessive loss of sperm) provides an example of a syndrome that received particular medical attention in the early nineteenth century. The establishment of hospitals for the insane marked out the treatment of madness as a separate medical specialism in the same way that voluntary hospitals did for other medical specialties during this period (Granshaw, 1989).

The authority of the hospital regime lay with the medical practitioner: patients were categorised by severity of illness and the curative force was physical manipulation.

'Moral treatment' provided a different and competing model. Rather than a *disease* of the mind, insanity was viewed as a varying state where there were periods of lucidity in which the person was sensitive to the surrounding environment. Since a disordered mind was seen as being a function of a disordered environment, restoration to 'normality' required the provision of an orderly environment.

William Tuke, the first English protagonist of moral treatment, designed the Quaker facility known as the York 'Retreat' to offer space where the patient had the opportunity to re-learn a normal life. The regime at the Retreat was designed to keep the disordering influences of society out and included a concern with the religion, social habits, lifestyle and activities of the patient. Since it was assumed that moral change and sanity emerged from social influences, mechanical restraints of all types were eschewed. A model of 'normal' life was implicit to the organisation of patient activity. Staff were to act as role models representing normality and interacting with patients to rejuvenate decency and normal social relationships through feelings of shame and guilt. Both of these models, but particularly moral treatment, fed a zeal for establishing a publicly-funded comprehensive asylum system. Asylums would restore the mad to health at the same time as relieving the financial burden on the community.

The Growth in State Regulation and Provision and the New Poor Law

The insanity legislation of the first half of the nineteenth century was part of increased state intervention in social problems more generally, where legislation included the Poor Law Act of 1834, the Factory Acts of 1833 and 1844, the Mines Act of 1842 and the Public Health Act of 1848. The force of government policy on lunacy was concentrated almost exclusively on its 'pauper' variant. Lunacy reform was linked to changes in the wider Poor Law system brought about by the 1834 Poor Law Amendment Act.

The major social, economic and demographic upheaval which industrialisation brought about had changed the nature of poverty. A second wave of enclosures (making common land into private) created a surge in the number of landless workers, rural unemployed and those dependent on the vagaries of the wage labour market. This increased the cost of poverty massively which the Old Poor Law was incapable of subsidising. Moreover, the informal familial structures which the Old Poor Law relief was designed to supplement were being eroded by mass urbanisation.

Certain enlightenment ideas were also detectable in the type of reform that the 1834 Act represented. In his *An Essay on the Principle of Population*, first published in 1798, Thomas Malthus suggested that poverty was inevitable in any society. Jeremy Bentham held the view that it was desirable to extend rationality and scientific principles to the social world with a view to obtaining a well-regulated and disciplined society and advocated the development of new types of social institution in which order could be sustained through discipline and surveillance. Bentham considered his design for an 'inspection house' to be suitable for a range of social institutions including schools, asylums, workhouses and prisons.

Whereas the 'old' Elizabethan Poor Laws provided a system of locally funded outdoor relief with which to support the poor, the new Poor Laws brought about a shift in values and type of provision. The 'old' Poor Laws were predicated on entitlement, whereas the New Poor Law stressed deterrence. The system of outdoor relief was replaced with institutionalisation based on the principle of 'less eligibility' or 'workhouse test': indoor relief had to be more distasteful than work available outside the workhouse.

Lunacy Legislation 1801–45

Between 1801 and 1844 there were 71 Bills, reports of select committees and inquiries relating to lunacy. The main government legislation leading to the establishment of a full-blown pauper asylum system provided by local authorities in England and Wales included the following:

1   The Select Committee of 1805 reporting in 1807 heard evidence about the appalling conditions in which many pauper and criminal lunatics were being kept by madhouse-keepers. The solution advocated was the building of large asylums (up to 300 beds) to ensure economies of scale. The 1808 Act the following year authorised, although did not compel, magistrates to erect publicly funded asylums in each county.

2   The 1815–16 House of Commons Select Committee undertook a two-year inquiry into the conditions in which pauper lunatics were kept. Much of the evidence was provided by the philanthropists who had developed an interest in lunacy reform. The shortcomings documented in the Committee's report included serious deficiencies, including overcrowding; a lack of attendants; an inappropriate mixing of types of patient; a lack of medical input; the overuse of mechanical restraints; poor physical health of patients; unwarranted detention; and inadequate certification procedures and inspection of private madhouses. Mistreatment was found to be prevalent in all types of institution. Yet, as Scull (1979, 77) points out, 'both the Committee itself and those who disseminated its findings to a wider public interpreted these revelations as proof of the need for more institutions', albeit ones under direct public control with an improved system of inspection and supervision.

3   The 1828 Madhouse Act repealed the 1774 Act and replaced it with a more rigorous system of licensing and visiting. The County Asylums Act passed in the same year required asylums to make returns of admissions and discharges to the Home Office and gave rights of visitation to the Secretary of State.

4   The 1844 Report of the Metropolitan Commissioners in Lunacy was able to provide systematic data of lunatics in all types of institutions for the first time. It conceded that the existing asylum system was a failure. The report showed that nearly half of all lunatics were being kept in workhouses and elsewhere. The fact that the number of admissions was not matched with discharges also indicated that the asylum had failed to realise its therapeutic promise in delivering cures for mental disorder. However, rather than abandoning this policy pathway, the government chose to reinforce the asylum system by the passing and implementing of the 1845 Lunacy Act. This act made the building of County Asylums compulsory and created a central regulatory body, the Lunacy Commission, which was authorised to carry out regular inspections of asylums.

Victorian lunacy reform

The Campaign for Lunacy Reform was led by an influential lobby of aristocratic philanthropists (such as Lord Shaftesbury), successful entrepreneurs and Quakers and Evangelists. Over and above a belief that medicine could cure insanity, the campaign focused on three issues:

1 the lack of asylum provision (charitable funding was limited)
2 harsh treatment of inmates by profit-seeking madhouse-keepers
3 the inappropriate placing of lunatics in workhouses

Although there is general agreement that philanthropic concern played
a central part in bringing lunacy to the forefront of government thinking and action, commentators suggest a variety of underlying motives.
Skultans (1979) considers that the philanthropists' campaigns were based
on benevolence and humanitarianism. Scull provides a more critical
account of the lunacy reformers, whom he viewed as being stimulated
by the less admirable values of evangelicalism and Benthamism, which
were imbued with dominant class interests.

According to Porter (1987), Georgian doctors had generally not been
interested in legal reform or lunacy policy. However, their early Victorian counterparts were deeply immersed in the shaping and making of
policy, and the relationship between the State and mad-doctors was of
mutual benefit. The attractiveness of a medical monopoly of madness
for the State seemed to rest on medical claims, which coincided with
the broad sweep of government thinking. Psychiatry could claim not
only that there was a rising incidence of mental illness that had to be
managed, but that investment in asylum-building was warranted because
of the promise of returning a large number of cures which would deliver
orderly and economically active citizens back into society. Thus, psychiatry made asylum-building an attractive option in the face of reticence
about the cost. In turn the acceptance of medical management by the
state reaped huge rewards for the mad-doctors. The establishment of a
comprehensive asylum system provided both a rationale for the confinement of lunatics in one place and an *opportunity* for the close scientific
scrutiny of odd behaviour, delusions and delinquencies necessary for
the development of a conceptual framework.

The 1845 Lunatics Act sounded the death-knell of lay administrators by awarding a monopoly of the running of institutions to medical
practitioners. The term 'psychiatry', which was introduced into British
medicine in 1846, is evidence of the link between the 1845 Act and
the emergence of a sub-specialty of medicine. Just over a decade later
(1858) the General Medical Act gave medical practitioners a monopoly
of control over illness. The same year the editorial of the *Journal of
Mental Science* (now the *British Journal of Psychiatry*) pronounced
that: 'Insanity is purely a disease of the brain. The physician is now
the responsible guardian of the lunatic and must ever remain so.' These
two sentences capture a political project of organised medicine which

was to last for over a hundred years: madness was a biological disorder and only doctors could oversee its management.

Accounts for the Rise of the Asylum

It is likely that the lobbying activities of lunacy reformers and medical practitioners were only responsible in part for the genesis and growth of mass confinement. The increase in lunatics was massive and far outweighed the growth in population. In the half-century following the introduction of the compulsory asylum system, the population grew by 80 per cent whilst the numbers of lunatics quadrupled (Scull, 1979).

That the population of asylums grew enormously is undisputed. However, there is far less agreement about the *reasons* for their growth. Most accounts view aspects of industrialisation as a causal factor in the process. The main features of industrialisation can be summarised as follows:

1 a rapid growth in population and geographical mobility
2 population and production mobility from rural to urban areas
3 a shift away from agricultural to factory-based production
4 a transformation of the social and political ordering of dominant ideas

Whilst these features were clear, the interpretation of their relative influence has varied. Below are some competing explanations offered.

(1) *A rise in rates of mental disorder*. This was the theory most popular in arguments for the establishment of asylums, particularly those made by medical practitioners. Some psychiatrists still argue that this was a dominant factor; it is assumed that, for example, 'schizophrenia' increased in incidence due to a viral infection in 1800 (Hare, 1988).

(2) *Humanitarianism and benevolence*. Another focus of analysis views the process as part and parcel of medical progress and an increasingly humane way of dealing with 'mentally ill' people (K. Jones, 1960).

(3) *Breakdown in familial and community support networks as a result of urbanisation*. Others see the growth of the asylum system as an inevitable result of the rise of industrial society. According to Mechanic (1969, 54), 'Industrial and technological change . . . coupled with increasing urbanisation brought decreasing tolerance for bizarre and disruptive behaviour and less ability to contain deviant behaviour within the existing social structure'.

(4) *The capitalist economy and an associated growth of psychiatric knowledge.* Scull claims that the mass segregation of madness 'can much more plausibly be asserted to lie in the effects of the advent of a mature capitalist market economy and the associated ever more thoroughgoing commercialisation of existence' (Scull, 1979, 30). Rather than the 'real' rates of mental illness amongst the population increasing, the proliferation of 'new' psychiatric classifications may have been important in drawing people into the asylum system. Insanity became 'such an amorphous, all-embracing concept, that the range of behaviour it could be stretched to encompass was almost infinite' (Scull, 1979, 238). According to Scull, the mad-doctors' motivation for the expansion of insanity classification was their increasing professionalisation.

(5) *Administrative changes in the operation of the Poor Law.* In the second half of the nineteenth century administrative convenience and financial incentives at local authority level accentuated the upward trend in the growth of asylum numbers. By 1867 the government was forced to act over the problems which had arisen with the implementation of the 1834 Poor Law. Most of those presenting for indoor relief were the 'non-able-bodied' poor, the sick, infirm and elderly, and it had never been the intention of the Poor Law Commissioners that the principle of 'less eligibility' be applied to this group (Cochrane, 1988). Moreover, despite the intention of the Benthamite reformers, outdoor relief still predominated for able-bodied paupers. (According to the Report of the Royal Commission on the Poor Laws in 1909, in the period 1871–9 the 'outdoor poor' outnumbered those in workhouses by 4.5 to 1. In 1896–1905 this proportion was reduced to 2.6 to 1.9.) During the latter half of the century, government attention focused on centring poor relief on the workhouse. Chronic lunatics in workhouses posed an impediment to such change. Many 'chronic lunatics' who remained incarcerated in workhouses did not fit the 'less eligibility' rule; also 'their detention in workhouses was objectionable on humanitarian grounds, and they were difficult to manage in workhouse wards' (Cochrane, 1988, 250).

The Triumph of Custodialism

The realities of the pauper asylum system bore little relation to the aspirations of the reformers. Although some asylums tried to copy the moral treatment regime, this was quickly abandoned, as were all other therapeutic regimes. Like the workhouses, asylums became large regimented institutions of last resort which, if anything, were more stig-matising. Although they were run by medical men, they failed to deliver the cures that a medical approach to insanity had promised.

A number of factors contributed to the custodial nature of the asylums.

1 *Certification* was a legal requirement for all inmates of public asylums, which acted as a deterrent to attracting cases likely to be 'curable' in that it encouraged early admission and prevented discharge.

2 The *physical design* and running of the buildings encouraged custodialism. Expensive, ostentatious asylum façades disguised a preoccupation with security (high perimeter walls and strictly controlled access) and the gloomy and drab prison-like interiors. Security concerns also came to predominate in the staff culture. (Busfield 1986)

3 There was also the *size of the asylum*. The earliest asylums had been built for less than 100 persons. By the end of the nineteenth century the average asylum contained 1000 inmates with some taking up to 2000.

4 The management of inmates was based on *the norms of the Poor Law*. Control was exercised through regimentation, routine and engendering passivity and dependence.

5 Finally, there was *little in the way of a therapeutic regime* in the asylums. The less physically and mentally able were confined to 'refractory wards', where restraint in padded cells and nocturnal sedatives were used. Some asylums used belts, straps and locked gloves to constrain patients and at the end of the century some returned to using mechanical devices (Tomes, 1988). Although the asylums were run by medical men, the superintendents of public asylums and their medical assistants assumed mainly an adminis-trative, rather than a therapeutic, role. The low wages and harsh conditions meant that the quality of the attendant staff was poor.

The culmination of custodialism in the latter part of the nineteenth century, which continued into the first decades of the twentieth, found expression in the 1890 Lunacy Act. Although critics of the asylums argued for trying to make them more therapeutic and less custodial by allowing admission without certification, early intervention and the boarding-out of the more chronic cases, the argument was lost. The 1890 Act is regarded as the triumph of a legalistic approach. Concen-trating as it did on wrongful certification and detention, it prioritised and protected the civil rights of those *outside* the asylum. Legislation

concerning the voluntary admission to hospital and a focus on treatment and therapy had to wait until well into the twentieth century.
But, as we shall see in the next chapter, it is a moot point whether or
not these changes which placed power and responsibility more firmly
in the hands of the medical profession represented a more enlightened
approach.

Whilst some commentators have talked of an oscillation between
medical and legal reform (Bean, 1986), another reading of the history
of asylums suggests a symbiosis of state (legislative and judicial) and
medical interests. Within this symbiosis the legal profession has never
achieved the same degree of recognition and power afforded by government to the psychiatric profession. Ultimately, so-called 'legalism' has
been administered, by and large, by the medical profession.

Was the asylum patriarchal?

Some feminist researchers have emphasised the patriarchal character
of psychiatry. Showalter's *The Female Malady* (1985) is frequently
cited in this field of inquiry. She argues that during the nineteenth
century women were overrepresented in the asylum system and that
madness was mainly a female condition. Moreover, she claims that
whilst furious male madness was the dominant cultural motif in the
eighteenth century, in the Victorian period madness was feminised in
artistic representations. This view has been challenged by sociologists
using official records from the time, that admission rates to the asylum
system were similar for men and women, but that because of differences in life expectancy more female lunatics accumulated. Women
were discharged more frequently than men and the latter were more
likely to die in the asylum than were women. In epidemiological terms
the incidence for madness for men and women was similar but the
prevalence was greater for the latter.

Showalter's emphasis on the cultural representations of madness being
slanted towards female images can also be disputed. Showalter emphasises
images such as suicidal Ophelia, crazy Jane or Kate and the violent
Lucia in Victorian art. These images were present but there were also
common cultural representations of male madness (the mad genius,
the criminal lunatic and masturbatory insanity). For sociologists such
as Pauline Prior psychiatry was gendered but contained a complex mixture
of attributions of both female and male irrationality and other
arrangement. For example the emphasis within Victorian psychiatry

was on the use of both restraint and male asylum attendants. These suggest that violent and disruptive behaviour were the organisational priorities in asylum work. The issue of gendered mental health work will be considered again later.

Industrial Fatigue and Shellshock: Mad-Doctors Found Wanting

In the wake of the 1890 Act psychiatry settled down as a paternalistic asylum-based discipline with little to show for itself as a medical specialism offering genuine cures for madness. The twentieth century was to witness a series of policy shifts which involved controversies surrounding the role of the mental hospital, psychiatric knowledge and the citizenship – or lack of it – of psychiatric patients.

The containment of pauper lunatics and the biological emphasis within psychiatry dominated the late-Victorian picture. The inmates of asylums were assumed to be mad because of faulty brains which were in turn a product of a tainted or flawed gene pool. This interplay between the incarceration role of the asylum and the bio-deterministic knowledge base of psychiatry was well suited for the regulation of a peacetime population. However, the First World War was to pose a different set of problems for government in relation to mental abnormality.

Industrial fatigue

The 1911 National Insurance Act was the first piece of legislation to provide for non-fee-paying patients. However, this was only for working men. With the outbreak of war in 1914 industrial output was at the expense of female labour. Moreover, the latter did not merely replace men in the factories, but literally doubled their efforts. In 1913 men worked between 48 and 55 hours per week in factories. By 1916 women were working 90 hours on average, with some exceeding 100 hours per week (Hearnshaw, 1964). Such was the concern about the physical and psychosomatic consequences of these conditions, which included anxiety reactions, miscarriages and exhaustion, that in 1915 Lloyd George set up the Health of Munitions Workers Committee (which was to become the Industrial Fatigue Board).

Other indications that the government after 1911 was taking the health and welfare of women and children (i.e., not just working men) seriously was that by the war's end the Maternal and Child Welfare Act (1918) was passed. This required local authorities to set up committees to review ante-natal and child medical services. A least some of the pressure for this focus on women during the war was the concern about the loss of male infants (Busfield 1986). The general point to note here, though, is that whereas in the pre-war period the focus was on purported genetic inferiority and its containment in institutions, government concern was now extending to stress conditions which were accepted to be environmental and whose victims were deemed to be honourable and genetically healthy (not 'degenerate'). This was one source of crisis for services based upon the bio-deterministic ideas and institutional containment. But the more salient pressure came from the mental problems of male combatants.

Shellshock

The crisis for Victorian psychiatric theory and practice created by shellshock is summarised well here by Stone (1985):

> The monolithic theory of hereditary degeneration upon which Victorian psychiatry had based its social and scientific vision was significantly dented as young men of respectable and proven character were reduced to mental wrecks within a few months in the trenches . . . Not only had shellshock effectively blurred the distinction between the 'neuroses' and 'insanity', but many chronically 'war-strained' ex-service men were, by the early 1920s, being transferred to asylums as inpatients.

The claim that these soldiers, proudly dubbed 'England's finest blood', were degenerate was logically impossible and tantamount to treason. This tension between explanatory notions of degeneracy and environmental stress became more evident as it was recognised that upper-middle-class officers were actually breaking down at higher rates than their subordinate ranks. As early as December 1914 reports from France indicated that 7–10 per cent of officers and 3–4 per cent of other ranks were suffering breakdowns. Consequently, as with the industrial fatigue problem at home, environmental theories were to be offered a place in the range of psychiatric theories. In the case of shellshock, this was to allow the emergence of Freudian-derived psychotherapy.

The scale of the shellshock problem is indicated by the medical records of the time, with 80 000 cases passing through army hospitals during the war and 30 000 being placed in psychiatric institutions. However, as Stone (1985) notes, this may be an underestimate given that many cases were given less stigmatising labels such as 'Disordered Action of the Heart'. Also, the distinction between 'normal' mental states and 'shellshock', under conditions of the daily filth and carnage of the trenches, could be arbitrarily determined by the extent to which local officers expected all under their command to 'tough it out'. Thus the more tough-minded officers would refer out fewer cases than more tender-minded colleagues.

If we consider the combined effect of industrial fatigue at home and shellshock on mainland Europe we see four features emerging which were to change irrevocably the face of twentieth-century psychiatric services.

1 Neurosis and not just psychosis was to become a focus of professional interest.
2 Environmental theories were to become a challenge to the bio-deterministic legacy of the Victorian period.
3 Services were to be organised on an outpatient as well as inpatient basis.
4 The gendered character of mental health shifted away for a while from that of asylum routines. The psychosomatic reactions of female munitions workers and the neurotic reactions of male combatants, rather than madness in either sex, became a focus for experts working outside the walls of the asylums.

The 1924–6 Royal Commission

Changing professional interests in outpatient psychotherapy with neurotic patients was evident in the new cultural legitimacy accorded to Freudianism. The first section of the British Psychological Society (the Medical Section) was set up in 1919 by shellshock doctors returning from the war. In the same year the British Psychoanalytical Society was formed. Prior to the war Freudian ideas had been rejected by the bulk of the British medical profession. In 1920, again with a Freudian character, the Tavistock Clinic was founded with its first honorary vice presidents being Admiral Beatty and Field Marshal Haig. The Ministry of Pensions set up a hundred outpatient treatment centres for shellshock cases returning from the war, and by the end of the war inpatient facilities were being used as intensive training centres for medical psychotherapists to practise on an outpatient basis. In the 1920s shellshock became a focus for both new forms of treatment approaches and a social administrative problem of compensation. As Stone (1985) notes, there were 100 000 such cases returning from the war, and so psychiatric disability, other than the lunacy identified by Victorian mad-doctors, had a double cost implication: from outpatient treatment facilities and from compensation claims.

This picture, with its emphasis on environmental causes of mental abnormality, meant that the legitimacy of asylum doctors in the eyes of both government and the public had been undermined in the war years. When the Royal Commission on Lunacy and Mental Disorder was set up in 1924, not a single asylum doctor was invited as a member. The stimulus for this commission, chaired by H. P. (Lord) Macmillan (1873–1952), was public concern about wrongful detention. In the post-war era public sensitivity about mental distress may well have been greater than in the pre-war period. After all, with all cases being certified under the 1890 Act, wrongful detention must have been rife at the turn of the century. The association between mental abnormality and a narrow band of 'riff raff' from what Marx called the 'lumpen-proletariat' – pauper lunatics – had now broken down. People with severe mental distress were visible from *all* class backgrounds in the wake of the war. Their treatment in the community in outpatient settings made this visibility greater. The expansion of the ambit of professional activity from pauper lunatics to include other social classes and forms of mental problem was both reflected in, and shaped, policy developments after the war. Accordingly, compassion about mental distress and concerns about softening the segregative emphasis of the 1890 legislation were prevalent.

The Commission reported in 1926 (HMSO, 1926) and its opening statement contained the following four emphases which demonstrate that its prime concerns were more theoretical than legalistic.

1 Mental and physical illness should now be seen as overlapping and not as distinct.
2 Mental illness typically has physical concomitants (even though they are not always readily discernible).
3 Physical illness typically had mental concomitants.
4 There are many cases in which it is difficult to decide whether physical or mental symptoms and causes predominate.

Thus, although asylum doctors were not *invited* on to the Commission, the *outcome* of its deliberations was remarkably consistent with the medical emphasis of Victorian psychiatry.

The Macmillan Commission's position was one which is still bedevilling modern attempts to make therapeutic law. On the one hand, there was an emphasis on the need for benign care, curative intent and consideration for the individual sufferer's needs. On the other hand, the emphasis on the need for the use of force in the case of mental illness actually requires the deprivation of liberty without trial: the removal of a fundamental civil right. The medicalisation emphasis of the 1930 Mental Treatment Act, in the wake of the Commission's 1924–6 report, thus incorporated such a contradiction. This legislation also marked a stepping-stone between the judicial emphasis of 1890 and the move away from the use of courts and towards even greater medical control under the 1959 legislation (see later). The 1930 Act, in accord with the Macmillan recommendations, extended the voluntary boarder system of the 1890 Act.

By 1930 the 1845 legislation's strictures about mandatory public asylums had installed a nationwide network of grand and extensive buildings near every major population point. England and Wales had 98 asylums which contained 120 000 patients (K. Jones, 1960). Only one new mental hospital was built in the inter-war period, at Runwell, Essex, but the Bethlem was rebuilt for the fourth time (Webster, 1988). The 1930 Act on the one hand signalled the end of a narrow segregation emphasis within British mental health policy, but on the other reinforced the medicalisation of mental abnormality. For this reason, it is hardly surprising that it did not in fact lead to a substantial alternation in asylum practices. A number of supportive findings and recommendations from the 1924–6 Commission's report worked in the interests of doctors. The prevention and treatment emphasis has been mentioned, but in addition there was the recommendation that doctors should be protected from being sued by patients or relatives (unless they were shown to be acting in bad faith).

Whilst most of the 1926 recommendations were converted into the 1930 Act, the ones which were *not* influential also reveal the intended or unintended support from Parliament for continued professional and asylum dominance in service organisation. For instance, Macmillan wanted information about legal rights for patients and relatives to be posted on hospital wards, but this was omitted from the 1930 Act. Likewise, the emphasis in 1926 on outpatients' clinics and observation beds in general hospitals (i.e., not asylums) was weakened and aftercare given over as a discretionary or 'permissive' duty for local authorities, with no central state finance being allocated for the purpose.

Thus, the first real opportunity to give formal state legitimacy to a policy of community- rather than hospital-based mental health services was lost with the passing of the 1930 Act. In 1929 the minority Labour government drafting the Act was in no position to guarantee resources for any new project. In the debate about the bill, community-based hostels were suggested twice by MPs but not incorporated into the Act.

Overall, the endorsement of most of the 1926 recommendations and the telling selective omissions led to the Mental Treatment Act emphasising asylum-centred services in the 1930s. Moreover, the original public sensitivities about wrongful detention in the early 1920s could not have been assuaged by the 1930 legislation. Whilst the 1890 Act was overly and overtly legalistic – 'nothing was left to chance' (K. Jones, 1960) – the greater medical emphasis of the 1930 Act meant that legal protection was weakened for patients and forced treatment become a mystification of, or rationalisation for, detention without trial. The legislators' trust in a medical-therapeutic ethos in mental health work bolstered professional power at the expense of the rights of patients.

In the inter-war period, for better or worse, the state was shifting its trust from judicial to medical regulation of mental abnormality in society. In fact, there were few empirical grounds for having confidence in the shift's beneficial value for those afflicted by mental distress. The hospitals of the 1930s were really little different from the Victorian asylums. They were merely the same buildings but with a new treatment rhetoric. In the early 1930s treatments were crude and somatic: chloral hydrate, cold baths, laxatives and paraldehyde. Somatic interventions had clear advantages for staff, in terms of producing a sedated and controlled inpatient population. But there was no evidence that they led to permanent cure. The one exception in this regard was the treatment of syphilitic psychosis ('General Paralysis of the Insane'), and even the prevalence and salience of this has been contested as being inflated (Prior, 1993).

The death rate in hospitals hardly inspired confidence either. Ramon (1985) reports that in the 1920s the number dying per year, around 9000, was virtually the same as those being discharged, around 10 000. This pattern of high death rates in hospital continued in the 1930s and beyond, indicating that the physical health of inpatients was very poor despite them living in a medical regime.

Other contributory factors to the mortality rate may have been the iatrogenic deaths from the new somatic treatments (insulin coma, psychosurgery and unmodified electroconvulsive therapy, or ECT) which were introduced during the mid-1930s, and the wholesale removal of tonsils and teeth (Clare, 1976). Any treatment involving coma or general anaesthesia had and has a predictable mortality rate. In the case of unmodified ECT, the absence of anaesthesia or muscle relaxants rendered the procedure even more dangerous to its recipients. As for hopes about a more benign and less restraining regime, in the mid-1930s around 90 per cent of patients were still detained in hospital compulsorily, despite the new emphasis on the voluntary patient.

The question begged, then, is that if the 1930 legislation, and service organisation in its wake, engendered little improvement for patients on the plight of Victorian lunatics, why did politicians hand over greater powers for the management of mental abnormality to hospital-based doctors? A number of factors can be suggested to account for this, many of which still apply today.

1   Mental patients had *no organised lobby* and so interest in and accurate knowledge about this group was weak among parliamentarians. In the debates preceding the 1930 Act the views of patients were hardly mentioned.
2   MPs would *gain few votes* by taking an interest in the topic of mental illness and even fewer if they supported patients' rights at the expense of increasing public fears and prejudices about madness.
3   Where interest was taken by MPs, some of these were *doctors* and so were directly representing a medical interest.
4   Finally, the perplexity surrounding irrationality and its causes meant that on the one hand MPs were unclear (as was everyone else) about what to make of mental abnormality, and, on the other, this ignorance induced a need to look somewhere for *authoritative answers*. Medicine obliged.

Putting these factors together, it is likely that the origins of this inter-war policy formation are to be found in confusion, ignorance and unintended consequences from legislators, not in a medical or legal conspiracy.

The Return of War and the Advent of the NHS

Despite the return to hospital-based somatic psychiatry in the inter-war period, when hostilities with Nazi Germany looked inevitable, the authority of asylum doctors was once more rejected by central government. In 1938 the psychoanalyst who was Director of the (outpatient) Tavistock Clinic, J. R. Rees, was appointed as Consulting Psychiatrist to the army. In 1939 Rees was elevated to the rank of brigadier and made head of the Army psychiatric services.

Another indication that psychological rather than somatic methods were in favour under war conditions was the introduction of psychometric testing. H. J. Eysenck, the incipient founder of post-war British clinical psychology, was appointed as a psychologist working with armed service patients at Mill Hill in 1942 (Pilgrim and Treacher, 1992). During the war years psychological tests were applied to armed service problems of selection, training, morale and rehabilitation from stress reactions (Privy Council Office, 1947; Morris, 1949; Vernon and Parry, 1949). At the outbreak of war, the Ministry of Defence was aware of the dangers of a repetition of the shellshock problem of the previous European conflict.

The pressures and demands of warfare stimulated a rush of quickly tried innovations from these psychologically orientated workers. As well as Eysenck developing the beginnings of psychometrics in clinical settings, small group psychotherapy and therapeutic community approaches were introduced (Jones, 1952; Main, 1957; Bion, 1958) which were to extend the range of therapeutic technologies available for both inpatient and outpatient work in later years.

This resurgence of psychological approaches to psychiatric work has to be placed in the context of the structural changes in health care organisation which the war facilitated. In 1929 the Local Government Act marked the end of the Poor Law. The workhouses and infirmaries were placed under the administration of public assistance committees. These were expected to secure accommodation for sick people, which facilitated the (uneven) development of local authority hospitals. These hospitals came under the jurisdiction, like other public health facilities, of the local medical officers of health. Thus there were the beginnings of public hospitals prior to 1939. Of course, the asylums had been a special case in this regard since 1845.

The war itself encouraged a further move towards a prototype of the NHS. The EMS (Emergency Medical Service) was set up, which co-ordinated the work of public and voluntary hospitals and had a regional structure. This also exposed the uneven standards of care, particularly in the smaller local hospitals. This range of quality was documented by a set of regional surveys of the nation's hospitals conducted by a voluntary body, the Nuffield Provincial Hospital Trust, in conjunction with the Ministry of Health. Because of the existing regulations surrounding asylums (and mental deficiency hospitals), these were not surveyed by the Trust.

The Hospital Board of Control was conscious of shortcomings of the existing mental health services during the 1940s but saw little point in surveying and reviewing their organisation in the absence of reforms of the 1930 Act. According to the chair of the Board this would require a review on the scale of a Royal Commission, so a case was made for leaving the old asylums out of any new plans for a national hospital service (Webster, 1988, 327). However, in 1943 the Board conceded the need for a closer linkage with general hospitals, and mental health services were at the last minute included in the 1944 White Paper on health.

Analysts of this period (Ham, 1985; Webster, 1988) point to a confluence of mounting pressures for a publicly-available, centrally-administered and centrally-financed medical service. (From its inception the NHS has been a misnomer. The main concerns of planners were about illness, hospitals and medicine rather than health.) A number of reports about hospital organisation prior to the formation of EMS and the Nuffield surveys had indicated concern about organisational incoherence and inefficiency, inadequate and inconsistent funding and variable standards (Dawson Report, 1920; Royal Commission on National Health Insurance, 1926; British Medical Association, 1938; Sankey Committee on Voluntary Hospitals, 1937). However, the BMA wanted a co-ordinated national service but based on an extension of the 1911 legislation on National Insurance rather than on general taxation.

Thus, although the British NHS is often cited as the main achievement of democratic socialism in 1948 (the 'jewel in the crown' of the post-war welfare state), it would seem that some version of an NHS was inevitable with these prefiguring reports and trends. This inevitability was reinforced by events in the war. In 1941 the coalition government had indicated its intention of setting up a national hospital service with the arrival of peace. In 1942 the Beveridge report on Social Insurance and Allied services included the recommendation of the formation of a national health service.

Notwithstanding the reluctance of the Board of Control to reorganise mental illness hospitals in line with the new NHS structure, after 1948 these hospitals were brought into line. However, in England and Wales this did not lead to a unified local administration of mental health services. Administration was divided between hospital authorities and local health authorities. In Scotland the old voluntary Royal Mental

Asylums were brought under the control of Regional Health Boards. Generally local authorities would delegate control to autonomous visiting committees linked to particular hospitals.

Thus the war had brought with it a major structural change with the formation of the NHS. However, the large Victorian asylums remained intact. Moreover, despite the re-emergence of psychological approaches with 'soldier patients' and the confidence this inspired after the war in sites such as the Tavistock Clinic and the Institute of Psychiatry, biological asylum psychiatry was soon to resume business as usual. The next chapter continues the story of post-war developments.

4

After the Second World War

Introduction

The previous chapter focused on the growth and dominance of the Victorian asylum system. This chapter summarises how, after the Second World War, the asylum went into a period of crisis for a variety of reasons, before declining. However, as we will note in Chapters 9 and 10, the professional routines of asylum-based psychiatry still remain powerful. Whilst the large hospitals have now been physically demolished or recommissioned for other purposes, the cultural impact of the asylum is still evident today. The story of the rise and fall of the asylum provides clues about the nature of this cultural inertia.

Another Royal Commission and the 1959 Mental Health Act

Throughout the first half of the twentieth century the number of beds in large institutions continued to rise, and peaked at around 150 000 in 1954, after which the numbers started on a downward spiral so that by 1992 this figure was reduced to 50 000. It is a common error to associate the 1950s with the so-called 'pharmacological revolution'. This account given by some social policy analysts (e.g., Martin, 1985; Jones, 1988) suggests that the beginnings of post-war deinstitutionalisation took place because of the technical breakthrough of neuroleptic medication. The myth was also repeated in the report of the House of Commons Social Services Committee in 1985 (see Goodwin, 1992, 17).

There is no evidence for this causal link. Neuroleptics were introduced in 1954 but the patterns surrounding discharge and inpatient

61

levels had already been set in prior years. Goodwin (1992) and Scull (1977) review the evidence about the impact of neuroleptics and conclude that although the drugs can control florid symptoms in some psychotic patients, they cannot explain changes in discharge policies implicating wider ranges of psychiatric patients with different symptomatology and diagnoses, who were not in receipt of neuroleptics. Neither can they explain why the de-institutionalisation took place other groups (elderly and mentally handicapped patients). At that time these were not seen as prime candidates for neuroleptic treatment, although later psychiatrists developed an enthusiasm for using the drugs on them. Also, whilst bed numbers were dropping in British hospitals before 1954 and continued afterwards, in some other European countries bed numbers actually *increased* after the drugs were introduced.

If the neuroleptics did not actually stimulate de-institutionalisation and the 'pharmacological revolution' was a myth, why did British asylums start to run down by the end of the 1950s? One explanation given within a Marxian framework is that the cost of institutional care became too great for a publicly-funded welfare system to accommodate within a capitalist economy. This 'fiscal crisis of the state' explanation (Scull, 1977) does not fit the 1950s because such an economic crisis was not salient at that point of post-war reconstruction. Spending on hospital services actually increased during this period. Also this is a crude economistic explanation, which is too global. It cannot account for cross-national differences within international capitalism, or for the differential policies for groups within nations.

By 1956, two years after the introduction of neuroleptics and at a point when Scull claimed fiscal constraints applied, there were 2000 more beds in use than in 1952 and 1000 more psychiatric nurses and 77 more consultant psychiatrists employed. However, then, and even a year earlier, there were signs that the government was recognising the problem of basing a mental health policy solely on traditional hospital-based psychiatry. As Goodwin (1992) points out, the middle of the decade was rife with conflicting messages from government. Hospitals were both supported and undermined at the same time.

In anticipation of elements of the 1957 Royal Commission and of the 1962 Hospital Plan, in 1956 the Chief Medical Officer argued that the future of services should emphasise community siting, an expansion of general hospital work and an upgrading of existing mental hospital facilities. It was not likely that there would be such an expansion on all three fronts; until then only the mental hospitals were resourced in the main. But what is significant is that the three elements were being mooted at all. They reflect changes in ideological forces, not economic factors. Why were community care and general hospitals cropping up again from the late 1920s as features of a debate about mental health? They surely must suggest that doubts were evident about a monolithic mental health policy being centred on the old asylum system. In other words, whatever fiscal concerns there were about the management of non-productive deviance by running down institutions, there were also pressures, and sincere aspirations, to improve the care of people with mental health difficulties. Wider cultural factors also contributed to the sounding of the death-knell of the old mental illness hospitals. After the Second World War, the image of the Nazi concentration camp haunted Western Europe.

In this context of mid-1950s contradictions, the Percy Commission was launched. This Royal Commission began in 1954 and reported in 1957. The tension between legal and medical power, dating back to the nineteenth century, was evident in its deliberations. The central issue here was the residue of certification from the 1890 Lunacy Act in the extant 1930 Mental Treatment Act. Legalists, such as the Magistrates' Association and the Justices Clerks' Association, emphasised to the Commission that certification should remain and that the non-medical court forum was still appropriate to make judgements about sanity and insanity. This position was also supported by the National Association of Local Government Health and Welfare Officers. However, whilst the Commission did not reject the need for compulsion, it went further than the 1930 Act in recommending that judgements about it should be left to clinical professionals. This excluded the final check on medical power by the courts, at least as far as civil or non-offender patients were concerned.

As with the 1926 Commission and the 1983 Mental Health Act, the 1957 Report accepted uncritically the formula of medicalising complex dilemmas about responding to madness and respecting civil liberties. This formula accepted that:

(a) cases of mental illness were validly and reliably identified by psychiatrists;
(b) the identification of mental illness automatically implied a *need* for treatment;
(c) the obligation to treat was so compelling that individual loss of liberty was warranted;
(d) psychiatric treatment was effective;
(e) the integrity of medical practitioners was beyond doubt.

One of the reasons why psychiatric legislation remains so controversial is that all five of the assumptions above are contestable and the shift from patient liberty to the medical right to treat remains disconcerting to many. However, the post-war legislation enacted in 1959 and 1983 by Conservative governments, but not challenged substantively by their parliamentary opponents, suggests that therapeutic law, with all its dubious premises, is accepted by politicians in principle.

The 1957 Report led on to legislation passed in 1959 which:

• emphasised medical treatment
• weakened remaining legal checks on medical discretion
• but also began to point to the demise of the Victorian asylum

The New Hospital Plan of 1962

It is not clear, even with this distance of time, whether the 1959 Mental Health Act was to be a salient factor in explaining one feature of the 1960s and 1970s, namely a series of hospital scandals. Possibly it was a background factor. The state had effectively handed over the manage-ment of mental abnormality lock, stock and barrel to a medically-managed regime and had washed its hands of any independent responsibility for the fate of individual patients. These scandals, which will be touched on again below, occurred in long-stay and old asylums. The latter were the scornful target of Enoch Powell as Minister of Health, who in 1962 announced his Hospital Plan, which was to have as much of an influence on psychiatric services as the 1959 Act.

Powell laid out his ideas for the Plan in the previous year at the Annual Conference of the National Association of Mental Health (now MIND). He viewed the Victorian asylums as outdated for the func-tions of modern psychiatric treatment and described them thus: 'There they stand, isolated, majestic, imperious, brooded over by the giant water tower and chimney combined, rising unmistakable and daunting out of the countryside.' However, once again the assumption held was that psychiatric treatment was effective (a sentiment repeatedly expressed by politicians sporadically since the beginning of the twentieth cen-tury). The intention was to phase out the old asylums and so only minimal finance was given for their upgrading (the third element pro-posed in 1956 by the Chief Medical Officer). Asylum beds were being reduced and were projected to be halved by the mid-1970s. A second major feature of the Plan was the combined use of community facilities and general hospital wards. The 1959 Act had a new clause which permitted patients to be admitted to any hospital facility, not just a mental hospital. This opened up the possibility of acute psychiatric admissions being diverted to general hospital units. A pincer policy of new acute units in general hospitals plus decanting chronic patients into community residential facilities would eventually make the old asylums empty and thus redundant.

Scull's (1977) cost-cutting thesis is persuasive in relation to this episode of policy formation. Powell and his Conservative government were keen to minimise public expenditure, and the run-down of the old expensive hospitals was a good opportunity to make fiscal savings. The need for run-down would increase over time with the progressive reduction in the cost-effectiveness of the asylums as patient numbers declined, since core maintenance costs would be the same independent of bed occupancy. Suspicion about Powell's commitment to a *positive* vision of a post-asylum world was reinforced by his emphasis on the short-term role of the district general hospital (DGH) units, but with little flesh for the bones of his predicted community facilities. Indeed, when eventually he produced in 1963 his follow-up plan (*Health and Welfare: The Development of Community Care*, Ministry of Health (1963)) this lacked the clarity and detail of the Hospital Plan. While most re-member Powell for his Hospital Plan, the follow-up document on community care is scarcely recalled.

If the 1959 Act had given the green light to medical power in the area of decision-making about patients, the 1962 Hospital Plan offered a different type of signal for psychiatry to increase its role in DGH units. These provided the perfect organisational opportunity to abandon the Dickensian image of psychiatry and move into the same organisational framework as other medical specialities. Psychiatry was, and arguably still is, the lowest-status medical branch. What ensued was a transfer of asylum theory and practice to DGH units and no new evidence of staff involvement with the communities of the patients they admitted (Baruch and Treacher, 1978).

What Powell's uneven policy prompt seemed to do was encourage a process of re-institutionalisation, from old to new hospitals, not community care. Whilst the rhetoric of community care was strongly present after 1962, no asylum was closed for many years. Hospital admissions increased during this period even though total inpatient numbers continued to decrease. The policy momentum for hospital run-down really only gathered pace in the subsequent decade.

The End of the Victorian Asylum?

The Victorian asylums were in crisis by 1970. A number of factors contributed to this. Inpatient numbers continued to drop. Central government was reluctant to finance large expensive hospitals which were due to be phased out. Psychiatrists were starting to enjoy the status advantages of new facilities in DGH units. Social critics and dissident clinicians, together dubbed 'anti-psychiatry' (Goffman, 1961; Szasz, 1963; Laing, 1967; Cooper, 1968), were attacking the dehumanisation of institutional psychiatry. Even social psychiatrists – who, in principle, accepted the legitimacy of psychiatric theory and practice – pointed to the anti-therapeutic impact of institutional life (Wing and Freudenberg, 1961; Brown and Wing, 1962). To compound this picture, the worst fears of these critics were being demonstrated by official inquiries into neglect and mistreatment in disparate hospitals.

Martin (1985) documents this series of hospital scandals. The fact that they occurred in both mental handicap and mental illness hospitals suggests that the responsible factors for a failure of care were organisational and not linked to patient variables (except for the unrewarding nature of chronic groups). The main source of personal degradation for patients was simply institutional life itself. At this point the organisational *raison d'être* of the old hospitals is worth restating: they existed to segregate burdensome or threatening deviance.

The sensitivities of inmates were always a secondary (and sometimes merely rhetorical) consideration. The complacency of policy-makers at this time about what was going on in the asylums is indicated by the cessation of the monitoring of activity in mental illness hospitals between 1959 and 1965. Data collection recommenced just before the public exposure of the string of hospital scandals (Davidge *et al.*, 1993).

It is not surprising, then, that large hospitals led to what Martin describes as 'the corruption of care'. Places ostensibly designed to care for people ended up betraying and mistreating them. The scandal hospitals, Martin reviews, demonstrate this phenomenon repeatedly. The common features of the places explain this outcome: they were closed systems unchecked by external corrective feedback. Life in the old 'bins' was isolated geographically and professionally. Wards were themselves isolated 'fiefdoms' within a large hospital setting. They permitted the privacy which is a prerequisite of neglect and abuse. Consultants visited their patients infrequently. The chronicity and 'refractory' nature of long stay patients made them unrewarding to work with and sometimes difficult to control. These factors together culminated in widespread mistreatment.

The response of the government to this crisis in the old hospitals system was to establish visiting teams from the Hospitals (now 'Health') Advisory Service (HAS), which was created in 1969. Members of visiting teams were drawn from a multi-disciplinary mental health background and therefore had been, or were, involved in directly providing services themselves. Reports of these visits acted in a limited way to bring about improvements in the quality of care by highlighting resourcing and staffing problems, and exposing institutionalised staff to scrutiny informed by a broader set of norms. Staff and management were forced to account for practices and conditions within the hospitals in which they worked. The HAS teams, however, suffered from the same deficiencies as previous inspectorates. They were unable to enforce any change and were limited to making recommendations with no direct access to resources. None the less, it is likely that the existence of the reports of these visits, which highlighted poor physical amenities and staff practices, contributed to the view that the old asylums had outlived their utility and needed to be replaced as a matter of urgency.

The HAS reports certainly carried some weight in drawing the attention of government departments to the problems of organising and managing mental illness hospitals. The Nodder Report (Department of Health and Social Security, or DHSS, 1980a) was the outcome of the considerations of a DHSS-initiated working group which was set up in order to examine these highlighted problems. The working group recommended the establishment of clearly defined management structures for mental health services, including the creation of district psychiatric services management teams and hospital management teams to provide leadership in the development of local services. The report also emphasised the need for clear objectives, standards and targets to be set, against which progress could be measured. Annual progress reports were another recommendation. Nodder underlined the importance of joint planning with local authorities and, in a departure from previous policy statements, stressed the desirability of the involvement of community-based groups and organisations, such as the Community Health Councils and voluntary organisations.

This may explain why there was a post-war sensitivity to the degradation risked in closed institutions. Given the other professional, policy and economic factors stacked against the old hospitals, their days were clearly numbered. However, whilst it was one thing in political and professional circles to condemn the degradation of the old hospitals, it was another thing to be able to claim that their closure automatically marked progress. Three difficulties were already apparent in this regard, which remain important agendas today and will be explored in later chapters: clinical professionals showed no sign of embracing community-sited interventions; a gross imbalance of resourcing had emerged between hospital and community facilities; and there were fiscal pressures on the British government to reduce even further its commitment to public spending. Labour politicians of the 1970s were uncomfortable, but also impotent, about a hospital-centred legacy (Busfield, 1986). The gross resource imbalance between health and social services reflected the problems which existed about constructing a genuine policy of community care. This difficulty was compounded by the difficulties affecting Western capitalism in the wake of the oil crisis which we pick up at the start of the next chapter.

It is in the 1970s, not the 1950s, that Scull's cost-cutting thesis is valid. But, even then, it gives undue emphasis to the single factor of economics. Within the economic constraints of the time, pressures and aspirations were still evident about improving services. Hostility towards the old hospitals in many quarters was real, as were aspirations to give 'the mentally ill' a better deal. None the less, if we put together the bias towards the funding of hospitals at the expense of community facilities alongside the wider constraint on public spending, then community care was a vulnerable policy. Whilst the prospect of closing the old asylum and re-siting acute psychiatric care in new DGH units was good, the prospect of a well-resourced community service for the person with long-term mental health problems was not.

Gendered Mental Health Work Revisited

In the last chapter we noted the discrepancy in accounts about gender and the asylum. We also noted that the Great War brought with it new forms of gendered concern, such as the psychosomatic toll of female workers and the shellshock suffered by returning male soldiers. By the final quarter of the twentieth century, women were consistently over-represented in psychiatric statistics. However, as with the caution about the gendered nature of Victorian psychiatry being complex and impli-cating men as well as women patients, so too with more recent times. Elsewhere (Pilgrim and Rogers, 1999a, ch. 3) we have argued that the overrepresentation of women in the mental health system is largely accounted for by the expansion during this century of the ambit of mental health work to include outpatient and primary care interven-tions. This has been associated with the greater diagnosis of neurotic

conditions, especially depression, in women, only part of which is referred on to inpatient facilities. When we look at the diagnosis of
schizophrenia in inpatient settings gender differences are not apparent,
but women are overrepresented there because of higher rates of depression. Another continuing factor which sustains gender differences
is the greater average life expectancy of women. This has meant that
mental health problems in old age during this century (including
depression and dementia) have been more prevalent in women.

An implication of these gender differences is that whilst men remain underrepresented, overall, in psychiatric statistics, they are
overrepresented in certain settings such as secure provision, which entail
more coercive regimes. Moreover, whilst from the mid-1960s to the
present day the trend has been for a greater throughput of both male
and female patients to open psychiatric facilities (i.e., an increase in
the frequency of admission and discharge), the increase in female admissions has been less than for men. This has led to a trend in which
the overrepresentation of women in psychiatric settings is declining.
For example, in 1980 the ratio of female to male admissions was 1.4
to 1. By 1986 this had dropped to 1.28 to 1, and it was 1.25 to 1 by
1989 (DH, 1989, 1992a).

However, in contrast to this shift in hospital admissions towards men,
the higher prevalence of female mental health problems in the community, in the context of poorly-developed community care, has meant
that services have not been developed to meet women's needs, especially in relation to the stresses involved in the caring role (Cobb and
Wallcraft, 1989). The question of gender will be considered again, but
in relation to the mental health workforce, in Chapter 5.

The Fiscal Crisis and Thatcherism

After 1979 successive Conservative administrations radically pruned
and restructured the public sector. Before 1979 there was a welfare
state; after that year there emerged a 'mixed economy of welfare',
which contained an engineered blend of public, private and voluntary
services. However, during the 1970s a Labour administration had struggled
with debt problems amplified by the OPEC oil crisis in 1973 and had
had to approach the International Monetary Fund for a loan. A condition of this arrangement was that public spending had to be brought
under control. And so a Labour government began a period of welfare
cuts even before Thatcher came to power in 1979. Offe (1984) has

noted that the crisis of the British welfare state can be viewed as endemic to any capitalist country which attempts to solve its social problems by the use of public finance.

These financial considerations put pressure on expensive institutions such as the Victorian asylum system, but the latter had in any case been losing their credibility since the mid-1960s. Thus the run-down of the old asylums gained momentum for both economic and ideological reasons. Indeed, whilst economic factors were influential, it is worth noting that asylum run-down, and the absence of new large institutions being commissioned, had become a global trend, independent of particular nation-state economic conditions. Sometimes a reaction against the large hospital and for new community developments was stronger in some capitalist countries during the 1960s and 1970s (e.g., the USA and Italy) than in others (e.g., Spain and Japan). What was clear, though, was that the overall trend was one of what has been variously called the 'desegregation', 'de-institutionalisation' or 'decarceration' of those diagnosed as being mentally ill.

Britain during the 1980s followed this global trend but pursued desegregation within a wider framework of Conservative social policy. Essentially the latter abandoned versions of Keynesian compromise in fiscal policies and opted increasingly for a mixture of privatisation and marketisation: that is, what were previously publicly provided services were now put out to tender and contracted in. At first, large public bureaucracies, such as the NHS, were only tinkered with (e.g., the privatisation of hospital cleaning services). Marketisation was the other government strategy applied later in the 1980s, with the application of an internal market (or 'quasi-markets') to the NHS.

What privatisation and marketisation had in common was the ideological assumption that market mechanisms would provide the most cost-effective or efficient method for limiting the fiscal burdens that a capitalist economy both created and had to tolerate. These burdens result from non-productivity (i.e., those groups of people existing outside the productive process). These include children, old people, those mentally or physically inefficient for work purposes, the short-term sick and the long-term disabled, and those who are able but simply not required. It is hardly surprising, therefore, that these groups became particular targets for government reform during the 1980s.

A third thread (in addition to privatisation and marketisation) which can be identified as running through government policy in the 1980s was managerialism. The strong presence of this trend (the NHS is now managed, not merely administered) itself marks a contradiction. The main ideological thrust of Thatcherism was a claim of 'rolling back the state' and letting a combination of market forces and individual choices and initiatives (such as charitable actions) determine the outcome and organisation of civil life. Thus, managerialism was not a necessary consequence of monetarism. Indeed, it indicated a bureaucratic, not a market, strategy to improve efficiency in the public sector.

Managerialism has reflected a political compromise for Conservative governments fearful of the electoral consequences of full-blooded privatisation of the NHS. If an internal market could be effected and managers installed, as in private companies, then the public sector could be run as a business. Making managers into purchasers of services pushed this logic even further. Compared to the more radical New Right thinkers in the USA (such as Spicker, 1993), Thatcher offered a substantial compromise with welfare. The former have sought to expunge 'welfare paternalism' from their society. Thatcher was a politician rather than an armchair ideologue, and so she had to confirm in practice what neo-Marxian analysts had already predicted: that capitalism could not live comfortably with the welfare state, but ultimately it could not live without it either.

Mental Health Services in the 1980s

The sketch of wider changes in the British welfare state provides many hints as to the fate of mental health services in the 1980s. However, some of these changes cannot simply be reduced directly to the triple impact of privatisation, marketisation and managerialism, and one of its main consequences, consumerism. In addition to the these factors, there were policy processes which had been set in motion earlier. For example, in the last chapter the consensus about de-institutionalisation was noted. With the crisis about the old asylums in mind, let us now consider changes in mental health policy in the 1980s under a series of headings which respond to the following four questions.

1 Why were the old hospitals vulnerable to closure?
2 Why, though, did a reliance on inpatient work continue?
3 What was the impact of a restructured welfare state?
4 What was the impact of legislative changes in the 1980s?

The rest of this chapter will deal with these questions.

Explanations for hospital run-down

Explanations for the trend of large hospital run-down and closure may be summarised under four headings.

● the introduction of new psychiatric drugs
● economic and fiscal determinants
● a shift from chronic to acute problems
● a shift in psychiatric discourse

The assumptions of what may be termed a 'pharmacological revolution' suggests that hospital run-down occurred because of the successful use by psychiatrists of major tranquillisers from the late 1950s onwards.

This model is problematic for a number of reasons. A drop in numbers in psychiatric hospitals in Britain actually began *before* the introduction of the drugs. In additional, hospital run-down emerged as a policy for a wide range of patient groups who did not receive the drugs (e.g., people with learning difficulties, elderly people). Also, the rate of hospital run-down did not accelerate after the drugs' introduction.

A final problem with the pharmacological explanation is that drugs are not always effective and discharged groups of psychiatric patients include those who are resistant to their symptom-reduction impact. We can only speculate that such a weak explanatory model emerged and was maintained because it suited the interests of the psychiatric profession which emphasised the purported 'revolutionary' impact of major tranquillisers.

Economic rather than pharmacological determinism has been emphasised by Scull (1977), who argues that after the Second World War governments increasingly struggled to contain the fiscal pressures of the welfare state. Given that institutional care or segregative control was expensive, the large hospitals could be eliminated to save money. Scull's model is not only economistic in its explanation but cynical and depressing in its political conclusion. He contends that the horrors of the asylum have simply been replaced by ones of a different type, placing patients between a rock and a hard place: 'the alternative to the institution has been to be herded into newly emerging "deviant ghettoes", sewers of human misery, which is conventionally defined as social pathology within which (largely hidden from outside inspection or even notice) society's refuse may be repressively tolerated' (Scull, 1977, 153).

Scull raises an important caution here about the social and personal impact of de-institutionalisation, which we return to in Chapter 10: the vulnerability of ex-hospital patients in the community. The fiscal pressure hypothesis fits poorly with the period of the 1950s and 1960s when the policy of de-institutionalisation was introduced (on paper if not in practice), and fits better for the 1970s and after. The latter has been a period which we have already noted was associated with stringent efforts on the part of both Labour and then Conservative administrations to contain welfare spending. Rather than services being cut back they have changed their focus from long-term residents to acute and primary care work. What is consistent with this interpretation is that acute psychiatric beds, although fewer in number than the prior volume of the old hospitals, consume most of the State's spending on mental health services. It is an interpretation which also fits with the recent reports which have emphasised the tendency of services to overlook or neglect the needs of people with long-term mental health problems existing outside hospital beds.

A variation on this theme of psychiatry becoming differentiated is put forward by Rose (1986) who argues that:

Rather than seeking to explain a process of de-institutionalisation, we need to account for the proliferation of sites for the practice of psychiatry. There has not been an extension of social control but rather the psychiatrisation of new problems and the differentiation of the psychiatric population ... The modern dispensation of psychiatry, far from being merely repressive or negative has constituted a new discipline of mental health. (Rose, 1986, 83–4)

Essentially, Rose's argument here is part of a wider critique of the work of Marxists such as Scull who have emphasised psychiatry as part of a state apparatus of social control and have advocated fiscal crisis arguments to account for de-institutionalisation. This alternative model places an emphasis not on central decision-making about service balance but instead on a *change in psychiatric discourse*. In other words, this approach maps shifts in psychiatric knowledge. Similarly Prior (1991) has argued that over time the object of interest of psychiatric practice has changed. He suggests that after the nineteenth century the new, more psychologically-orientated discourse within psychiatry (a mixture of psychodynamic and behavioural theories) fitted less and less well with the old large institution. We have argued elsewhere (Pilgrim and Rogers, 1994) that these newer sociological accounts, which shift our attention away from government policy and towards a new psychiatric eclecticism, have been useful. They are not limited to the biological and hospital focus of, say, Scull's work. However, as we argue recurrently in this book, services may not be limited to this focus but they are *dominated* by it. Nonetheless an important differentiation of policy in the 1980s was the separation of acute and chronic services. Ramon (1985) pointed out that at the time of writing there had not been the full closure of a single Victorian asylum in Britain. However, because in the period after that old hospitals were indeed run down and closed, the configuration of mental health services included:

(a) the remaining unclosed large hospitals, which were often in poor repair and containing anxious or demoralised staff (who were themselves often institutionalised);
(b) newer acute inpatient services, which varied from purpose-built units in new general hospitals to wards of older general hospitals designated for psychiatric purposes;
(c) a mixture of community residential facilities (hostels, group homes, private bedsits and other tenancies, nursing homes);
(d) community mental health centres and day centres run by both the NHS and social service departments;
(e) regional secure units;
(f) the special hospitals.

Such a mixed picture of provision demonstrates that the term 'de-institutionalisation' fails to capture accurately what was (and still is) happening. Services were still dominated by forms of hospital organisation and so it is more appropriate to think of a process of *re-institutionalisation*, rather than full-scale and proper de-institutionalisation.

The inertia of hospital dominance

On the face of things the last decade has witnessed a decline in the pre-eminent position of the hospital in Britain, as in most other countries. Thirty-five 'water tower' hospitals closed by 1990. Additionally, the number of patients in large hospitals also halved from an average of 468 patients per hospital in 1986 to 223 per hospital in 1993 (Davidge *et al.*, 1993). However, most of this activity has occurred since the end of the 1980s (over half of these hospital closures occurred in the four years prior to 1993).

Notwithstanding the diversification away from large NHS hospitals to a wider range of provision, including local authorities, and the voluntary and private sectors, the shift of emphasis in psychiatric services was not predominantly from the old asylums to community facilities but from old to new hospitals. This is not say that community facilities failed to expand during the 1980s: it is simplistic to argue (as some critics did at the time) that community care was non-existent. It is, however, fair comment that the vision of community care, implied in the 1930 Mental Treatment Act and advocated by the Royal Commission of 1957 and in the Powell legislation in 1963, was still clouded throughout the 1980s by the inertia of hospital dominance. The closure plans for the remaining 89 hospitals open in 1993 shows the reluctance to make a clean break with the old hospital sites even with the accelerated rate of run-down evident at the beginning of the 1990s. A survey in the early 1990s (Davidge *et al.*, 1993) indicated that in less than a quarter were there plans for the closure and disposal of the whole hospital site. The intention, in over half of the cases, was to close the main building but retain some of it for mental health units on site.

It will be remembered from the last chapter that the Hospital Plan of 1962 had more of an impact than the Community Care Plan a year later. It was clear from the early 1960s onwards that planners and medical lobbyists in each locality were inclined to reform and adapt *hospital* facilities rather than innovate around community support services for home-based patients.

Hospital dominance was also evident in the way in which day care was offered to patients. For example, only 9000 new day places became available between 1975 and 1985 and these were mainly on hospital sites (Audit Commission, 1986). By the late 1980s, 85 per cent of government funding of mental health facilities was spent on hospital services (Sayce, 1989). By 1987 there were 49 CMHCs (Community Mental Health Centres) in existence, with 44 more planned. Whilst the stock of CMHCs expanded rapidly, because they started from a low base their absolute numbers and levels of funding remained small compared to psychiatric inpatient facilities by the late 1980s.

Tomlinson (1991) describes how the sources of this hospital focus, rather than community focus, were formalised by the DHSS in 1968 when the DHSS commissioned a development project in Worcester to demonstrate how a large asylum could be replaced systematically by other facilities. Powick Asylum was to be phased out and replaced by DGH and hostel facilities at Worcester and Kidderminster, with day facilities in Malvern and Evesham.

The Powick run-down programme encountered problems that were often to reappear during the late 1980s in other places: the tendency to leave the most difficult chronic patients until last as a discharge priority; staff morale problems in a declining institution; and the deterioration in the fabric of buildings that were to be shut. Powick closed eventually in 1989. A positive finding from research on the Worcester project was that the day facilities opened to support the closure programme were endorsed by service users as boosting confidence and warding off loneliness. Later research on users' views of services also suggested that non-hospital services are highly valued (Rogers, Pilgrim and Lacey, 1993).

The assumptions behind the Worcester development project reflected deep-seated difficulties about local and national politicians being able to think beyond the bricks and mortar of hospitals. The fact that there was such a strong rhetoric from Labour and Conservative government sources over a 20-year period about community care only highlights this picture. The selective attention to the legislation in the early 1960s (spotlighting the DGH and marginalising the need for non-hospital facilities) was evident in the mindset of planners in both the 1970s and 1980s. Part of this was probably a function of the political reliance on professional advice. As key stakeholders, psychiatrists are not only clinicians who lobby government via their Royal College (which was set up in 1971), but they also dominate the civil service roles in the DH which develop mental health policy and advise ministers.

Another factor which may have induced inertia about hospital dominance is the caution and conservatism from British politicians about the containment of deviance. The appeal of segregation to politicians is obvious: people who are disruptive, difficult or frightening can be dealt with in hospitals. The regime separates these people from those around them who are discomforted by their presence. The non-mad are in the majority and the majority cast votes in elections. The circle that politicians have to try and square is that segregation is both wanted and distrusted by the general public. Madness in the street and the home can be swept into hospital, but what if this strategy is both ineffective and offensive in its response? It is not an uncommon experience for ordinary citizens to want madness removed from their presence whilst fearing for their own arbitrary incarceration. The 1983 Mental Act, to be discussed below, responded to this contradictory demand.

Health and social services in turbulence

Whilst the bias towards hospital services can be seen as a function of cultural inertia in Britain during the 1970s and 1980s, a wider concerted restructuring was to some extent to override these forces from the past. In doing so a number of contradictions were set up and problems posed for a variety of stakeholders. Politicians had to face awkward questions about the non-medical functions which the old hospitals had served, such as social control and that of *accommodating* one group of people outside the productive process. By unleashing consumerism, via marketisation, the government offered hope to people whose views were previously ignored by service providers: psychiatric patients.

Psychiatrists and other mental health professionals were to find themselves victims of a wider attack by government on professionals. Professional elites, such as doctors and lawyers, are traditionally conservative groups (with a small and large 'c'). And yet throughout the 1980s the Conservative government systematically challenged or attacked the power of these elites. This was an ideological symptom of undermining the power of welfare 'bureau professionals', but it also reflected a more general attack on the authority of professionals. This authority had previously signified a form of power which was autonomous from the state. Despite the rhetoric of 'rolling back the state', Thatcherism was set upon reining in and controlling forms of authority which had been outside central government.

During this period local government was similarly undermined and dominated from the centre. Strict limits on local spending were instituted and the traditional powers of local education and health authorities reduced. By the end of the decade the 1990 NHS and Community Care Act (see below) was to impose what was labelled as a 'poisoned chalice'. Local authorities were to be made responsible for community care but were not given autonomous powers or guaranteed finance for the task. In addition, throughout the 1980s, public services were converted systematically into business-type organisations.

A centrally-driven and controlled policy of managerialism was a self-fulfilling prophecy from government in the early 1980s. If a businessman is given the task of reviewing the efficiency of public organisations, he will inevitably offer business solutions in response. Such was the case with the first Griffiths Report.

A new legislative framework

After 1979 there were two major pieces of legislation relevant to the
focus of this book. The first of these was the 1983 Mental Health Act,
and the second the 1990 NHS and Community Care Act. In the case
of the 1903 Act, this has to be seen as part of a review process, which
preceded the wider welfare restructuring imposed by Thatcherism.
Consequently, it was part of a pattern recurring in Britain every 20 or
30 years throughout the twentieth century: for instance, the Acts of
1930 and 1959 and their prior Royal Commissions. Such reviews have
considered very similar issues.

1   How is mental disorder to be defined?
2   Who should have the power and responsibility to respond to men-
    tal disorder?
3   What should be the balance between the right to be left alone and
    the right to be treated, especially when the latter is recognised by
    others but not by the mentally-disordered themselves?
4   Which aspects of citizenship should be legally protected for men-
    tally disordered people?
5   Under what circumstances should a person be removed forcibly to
    a psychiatric facility, and what rules should govern their detention
    and discharge?

Given the recurrent nature of these types of questions, which were
considered in the review leading up to the 1983 legislation, the Act
was a separate development from the wider social and health policy
changes that were being effected after 1979. The impact of the Act
was small in comparison with these other events. An extract from the
parliamentary debate prior to the introduction of the Act summarises
its purpose:

> that except in particular circumstances people should not be admit-
> ted to detention for treatment in hospital if their condition is
> not treatable; the provision of much more frequent access to mental
> health review tribunals; the more stringent regulations of the use
> of treatment without the consent of the patient; the institution
> of a special health authority, with particular responsibility to over-
> see the powers to detain and treat patients under the Act; the institution
> of interim hospital orders, the power to remand to hospital for
> assessment; and I think the limitations of the powers of a guardian

to apply only to people over 16 years of age. (Lord Elton, *Parliamentary Debates*, 1 December 1981, 935)

The Act did not endeavour to introduce new principles but to alter those of the 1959 Act and to improve administration (Bean, 1986). Its main achievement was the formal codification of existing professional roles and practice in relation to the compulsory detention of patients (e.g., the requirement for social workers to interview in a suitable manner). It had little or no direct relevance for informally detained patients, but it did introduce some new protections for those detained forcibly ('formal patients'). This included the right to lay or legal advocacy at Mental Health Review Tribunals, which could be applied for under the legal aid scheme, and the delegation of powers of discharge for patients who, under the 1959 legislation, could only be released by the Home Secretary.

Voting rights were introduced for informal patients only. Even these were nearly absent from the legislation. A Labour amendment was put forward for the preceding Mental Health (Amendment) Act 1982 to ensure the voting rights of all patients. Some Conservative MPs with mental hospitals in their constituencies wanted no voting rights for patients at all, but the government conceded a compromise, which remained highly discriminatory. Detained patients were not allowed a vote and informal patients can vote only if they complete an application without assistance. This subjected them to a literacy test which non-patients do not have to encounter at an election. In other respects the Act introduced new restrictions on patients' liberties. For example, under Section 5, registered mental nurses were given 'holding' powers forcibly to detain 'informal' patients in lieu of an assessment for compulsory admission.

The essential weakness of the 1983 Act was that it was overly concerned with individual rights. It had no direct implications for service organisation and the collective rights of patients. However, these very weaknesses meant that *the failure* of some aspects of the Act highlighted expectations of good care. For example, Section 117 for the first time raised the question about the duty of aftercare for discharged patients. Because this Section exists, it has allowed critics of inadequate services to draw attention to failed expectations about community care. A second unintended consequence for services has been the weakness of the Mental Health Act Commission (MHAC), the main structural innovation of the 1983 Act, in preventing the emergence of scandals and ridding the mental health system of bad practice.

The MHAC is a special (regionalised) health authority, which has a duty to check on the proper application of formal sections (detained patients). This watchdog role is limited to investigating individual complaints and so offers no solution to systemic difficulties. The first ten years of the MHAC witnessed a public acknowledgement of its failure to deal with neglect and brutality whilst, arguably, raising the expectation that civil liberties were now to be protected by such a statutory body. The most pointed example of MHAC failure was offered by the Blom-Cooper team investigating complaints of mistreatment at Ashworth Hospital (DH, 1992). The three-person team included both the Chair and the Vice Chair of the national MHAC and they conceded that the Commission had failed where investigative journalists (the *Cutting Edge* programme on Channel 4) had succeeded in exposing bad practice. Nothing had changed since 1980, when another television documentary had exposed brutality at Rampton Special Hospital. It seemed that with or without an MHAC, mistreatment was happening in closed isolated hospitals and a watchdog could not even be relied on to detect, let alone correct, such events.

When introducing an early analysis of the 1983 legislation, Bean described the new Mental Health Act as:

> part of a change worldwide which seeks to reduce the paternalism of an earlier age, to identify the rights of the individual patient, and to reduce (albeit marginally) the power and prestige of the psychiatric experts. Of course not everyone would welcome such changes but, in my view, they represent something of an advance, if only because the legislation produces doubts where once there was certainty, and shows that there are other ways forward even if those ways sometimes appear unclear. (Bean, 1986, 14)

However, looking back from today's perspective, we would conclude that the 1983 Act has been flimsy in its impact on service improvements. Evidence of the mistreatment of patients at the hands of psychiatric professionals has continued, and the legalistic and individualistic nature of the Act has been inadequate in the face of wider structural changes in health and social services. It has not reduced the rate of compulsory admissions, and it has raised, but not provided the means to meet, expectations of better treatment and improved patient rights (Rogers and Pilgrim, 1989). As a piece of legislation it also appears to have lost its relevance far sooner than previous mental health legislation. Its concentration on compulsorily detained patients in hospital, at a time of the rapid hospital closure programme, has meant that little more than a decade after its introduction the government was forced to consider new legislative measures. The latter ('supervised discharge') was introduced to manage and treat patients in a community context. (Even more recently, in 1999, the government started a process of 'root and branch' review of the 1983 Mental Health Act to ensure more efficient social control in the community in the future: see Chapter 12.)

The weak impact of the 1983 legislation can be contrasted with the 1990 NHS and Community Care Act. This was a crucial piece of legislation in a number of ways. First, it established a framework of service organisation for the four constituent countries of the UK (previously England and Wales had had separate legislation from Scotland and Northern Ireland). Second, it explicitly drew together duties across health and social service boundaries. Third, it was a catch-all piece of legislation which set out duties for several client groups. Prior mental health legislation in both 1959 and 1983 was not compatible with wider health reforms (such as the 1948 NHS Act). Thus, mental health law in Britain has been grafted on as an addendum to other relevant legislation, which has weakened both its remit and impact (Rogers and Pilgrim, 1986). The building blocks of the community care component of the 1990 Act originated in the review in 1988, *Community Care: An Agenda for Action* (HMSO, 1988). The Griffiths Report (as it was also known) provided an official endorsement of the notion that community care should be directed towards obtaining the best quality of life possible for people leaving hospital. The report outlined the principles needed to assure the success of the policy in the future by securing the following:

(a) appropriate services provided in good time to people who require them the most;
(b) the principle that people receiving help will have greater choice and say in what is done to assist them;
(c) help should be directed at allowing people to stay in their own homes for as long as possible, with nursing home and hospital care being reserved for those whose needs cannot be met in any other way.

The Griffiths vision was embodied in the 1989 White Paper, *Caring for People* (HMSO, 1989), and, with the exception of the recommendation that a minister should be designated with special responsibility for community care, subsequently translated into the 1990 Act.

The new Act involved:

- local authorities taking the lead in community care
- a duty of individual needs assessment and care management to deliver packages of care which would enable people to live at home
- Community Care Plans being drawn up in consultation with local people, either separately or in conjunction with health authorities
- 'arm's length' inspection units being set up to regulate standards in the 'independent' care sector and more effective complaints procedures in social services
- the separation of commissioning (purchasing or contracting) and providing functions (although unlike the case in the NHS this is not obligatory)
- the retention of responsibility for community health services by the NHS

Until May 1994, the last point meant that community mental health service planning was the responsibility of Regional Health Authorities. Since then, this power has been devolved to local commissioners of services for NHS authorities or Trusts. Regional Health Authorities were replaced in 1996 by regional outposts of the NHS Management Executive. Their role switched to monitoring services and facilitating service development.

Despite the radical implications of the 1990 NHS and Community Care Act, the debate about its impact was lopsided. The NHS part was the focus of considerable controversy, whereas the community care tag attracted less interest. Carpenter (1994a) suggested that public and academic interest was lukewarm because:

> The NHS reforms are seen by politicians, public and the media alike as something that will happen to 'us'. Will I have to travel to a distant hospital for treatment? Will my doctor be forbidden from prescribing a drug I need because of its expense? By contrast, community care is something which happens to 'the other' who might be pictured favourably as a deserving elderly or disabled person, or less favourably as a socially disruptive or even dangerous mental service user. Either way, it is only regarded as important to the extent that it might impinge on 'us' as either threat or burdens. Thus community care has not been given the priority it merits, because it is seen as an issue affecting others who are less socially and economically important, and who are not politically well placed to challenge this ascription. (Carpenter, 1994a, 20)

Carpenter goes on to identify a series of potential problems with the legislation which proved to be valid in the period between 1991 and 1997.

1   The transfer of funding from social security to community care local budgets was cash limited. Local authorities could not necessarily respond positively to needs once assessed.
2   A shift from hospital to community care and from expensive to cheap or unpaid care labour represented a form of 'dumping', disguised as demedicalisation and empowerment.
3   There was a limited emphasis on rights for community care clients; for example, community care was not identified as a right in the Citizen's Charter.
4   There were difficulties in shifting beyond a rhetoric of user involvement and empowerment.
5   Separate rather than seamless services were caused by splits and fragmentation of agencies: health/local authority/social security. This had the effect of making rehabilitation more difficult as the successful settlement of people in the community was only achieved by the health care system approaching other systems in order to accomplish the designated central government task of hospital closure (Bean and Mounser, 1993).
6   Managerialism had a limited impact in promoting cost-effectiveness when faced with inaction on other fronts which affected mental health, such as unemployment, poor housing, homelessness and discrimination. These implied a wider social policy framework to improve the quality of life and citizenship of community care clients, rather than merely increasing the efficiency and quantity of current (largely secondary and tertiary) services.

The 1980s: An Overview

The impact of unbroken Conservative government between 1979 and the early 1990s demonstrates a complex picture associated with an inertia about shifting from hospital-dominated to community-based support for people with mental health problems. When reflecting on this inertia, Beardshaw and Morgan (1990) identified five main difficulties, some of which still apply today.

1   Inter-agency collaboration is complex and often inefficient. Different parts of the system (NHS, social services, voluntary and private

sectors) have different ideologies and priorities. The aims of, say, inpatient providers will be different from those seeking to emphasise community mental health facilities. The translation of the ideals of documents such as the Griffiths Report often fell short because, as Bean and Mounser (1993, 25) pointed out, insufficient attention was given to the way in which the disparate systems providing aspects of community care operated in reality: 'Too often the various systems such as the benefits system, or the housing system, or the employment system, or the education system, work in isolation, follow their own codes and regulations, are in practice inflexible and work mutually to exclude each other.'

2   Mechanisms for effecting the shift of finance from hospital to community care were inadequate. Monies were lost following hospital closure for mental health facilities. If local authorities spent too much on building up community facilities, they were penalised by central government. Bridging funds for the transition between large hospital provision and alternatives were not made available.

3   The funding of private home placements by social security funds created a perverse incentive to generate mini-institutions in the community (rather than a range of ordinary living options).

4   Funding and educational innovations to equip institutionalised staff to work in community settings were inadequate.

5   Fear of innovation and failure and an attachment to traditional working practices on the part of planners and providers were evident. These features had been identified by the World Health Organisation (WHO) in 1977 as being the greatest impediment to improving mental health services.

The constraints and opportunities imposed by policies during the 1980s, characterised by privatisation, marketisation and managerialism, altered the way in which people of all political persuasions argued about improving mental health care. The opponents, as well as the advocates, of the long-serving Conservative administration reflected carefully on the vested interests of service providers, as well as on the best way to allocate restricted funds. It is for this reason that the opposition parties had to engage with arguments about user-empowerment and citizenship. In the past, finance alone had tended to dominate debates. The days when politicians took at face value what clinical professionals advised about planning services had passed. In Chapter 12 we examine the degree to which the Conservative legacy of 1997 was adapted and modified by an incoming Labour government.

Part III

Post-Institutional Developments

5

The Mental Health Professions

Introduction

Mental health professionals are stakeholders in policy development at a national level and in its implementation in particular localities. Policy determines professional activity, but professional values and views shape policy. Most of this chapter is about the dialectical relationship between professionals and their policy context. Eleven case studies are provided to illustrate this point about embodied mental health policy. We will cover the following:

1 the importance of expertise: the case of professional power/ knowledge
2 professional adaptation to policy shifts: the case of marketisation and its demise
3 agents of the State: the case of mental health law
4 the limits to professional autonomy: the case of self-regulation
5 the inertia of the asylum: the case of psychiatrists
6 in the wake of 1948: the case of clinical psychologists
7 breaking with the asylum tradition: the case of community mental health nurses
8 occupational substitution: the case of approved social workers
9 the threat to professional dominance: the case of the police and mental health work
10 inter-disciplinary work in flux: the case of primary and community care
11 the workforce as a mirror of wider society: the case of gender and class

The Mental Health Workforce as Embodied Policy

At the start of this book we drew attention to the importance of understanding policy as outcomes. One way of illuminating the processes
which mediate policy intentions and actual outcomes 'on the ground'
is to examine the activity of professionals. The latter embody political
dynamics. They pursue their own interests. They obey, resist or adapt
to the directives of politicians and civil servants. When policy is reviewed
and changes, professional groups are energised to influence the future.
The nature of mental health services is determined in large part by the
activities of specific professional groups alone and in interaction with
others. Below we give a series of examples which highlight these points
about embodied policy.

*The importance of expertise: the case of professional power/
knowledge*

The knowledge produced and used by professionals is not composed
of static entities divorced from policy formation processes; rather, professional ideas about the nature and treatment of mental health problems
impact on policy formation which in turn feeds back into professional
knowledge. For example, the differentiation of services for different
groups in the nineteenth century is related to different notions about
emotional and intellectual deviance. Prior to the 1890 Lunacy Act an
elaborate network of asylums had been built (see Chapter 3) which
contained 'aments', now known as people with learning difficulties or
disabilities, as well as 'dements' or 'lunatics'. As 'mental illness' and
'mental handicap' came to be seen as separate specialisms with distinct bodies of knowledge, so these were distinguished from one another
in policy legislation and provision.

The advent of community care policies has also heralded changes in
the conceptualisation of disease categories within psychiatry, which
have made the task of detecting and managing madness in non-
institutional settings by psychiatry easier. New models of schizophrenia
began to emerge. Positive symptoms which were once important in
deciding whether hospitalisation should occur are now displaced by an
elevation of the importance of so-called 'negative symptoms' (Andreason,
1989), because these reflect deficits in the patient's capacity to partici-
pate in ordinary social existence in community settings.

Within this discursive shift from positive to negative symptoms,
'schizophrenic' behaviour, which fails to meet criteria of self-motivation

and self-surveillance within a domestic or public context, is emphasised. Negative symptoms, such as 'avolition [lack of will] . . . manifests itself as a characteristic lack of energy, drive and interest', which often leads to 'severe social and economic impairment' (Andreason, 1989). Accordingly, psychiatrists now recognise aspects of a 'schizophrenic's' personal life which he or she is deemed not to be able to manage by him- or herself. Such problems include: irregular attendance at work, carrying out employment and domestic tasks in a disorganised and half-hearted manner, the lack of the pursuit of pleasure ('anhedonia') and a lack of interest in sex.

Professional adaptation to policy shifts: the case of marketisation and its demise

The 1990 NHS and Community Care Act changed the traditional territory of the mental health professions. The practical impact of this lasted between 1991 and 1999 when the 'internal market' was introduced, but was then displaced by Labour's legislation. An example of this can be seen in the impact of the purchaser/provider split. This entailed a number of professions vying with each other for access to receive referrals. Clinical psychologists now regularly accept referrals from GPs and may be commissioned as the providers of counselling or psychotherapy services. Two decades ago psychiatrists had a virtual monopoly of control over access to, and treatment of, patients, which constrained the autonomous work of subordinate professions such as clinical psychologists (Goldie, 1977).

Local management of finances by health agencies may also substantially change the numbers and influence of certain professional groups. Two examples illustrate the point. First, there may be substitution of one expensive profession with a cheaper one. Psychiatric nurses are cheaper to employ than psychiatrists. However, they can perform many of the same functions and so they may grow in both numbers and power at the expense of the former superordinate profession. However, some recent reports about mental health services have suggested that the skill mix in the work of community mental health nurses (CMHNs) is not cost-effective and CMHNs may themselves face challenges to their occupational territory from care assistants or community support workers.

Second, the government's 'fundholding' initiative between 1993 and 1997, which allowed GPs to buy services in addition to their traditional role of providing services, increased the role of primary care workers. GPs bought counselling services from non-psychiatric professionals because they were popular with patients, assigned mental health work to practice nurses, and substituted hospital psychiatric outpatient sessions for practice-based alternatives. GPs preferred these arrangements as they had control over the employment of staff and services rather than being placed in a traditionally subordinate position to liaison or hospital psychiatry.

Education is another way in which governments intervene in the mental health labour market. For example, the sanctioning of Project 2000, through the United Kingdom Central Committee (UKCC), engendered a different type of training for psychiatric nurses in comparison with the previous Registered Mental Nurse course. The government's 'White Paper 10' also set nursing on a path entailing all future mental health nurses being educated in universities. Previously, training was mainly in colleges of nursing, which were under the auspices of health authorities.

Agents of the State: the case of mental health law

Unlike other health workers, the mental health occupations also regularly carry out a social control function, which is governed by legislation in relation to both the civil compulsory detention of patients and the assessment, treatment and detention of mentally disordered offenders, under various sections of the 1983 Mental Health Act. A rare example of this in another field is the 1948 National Assistance Act, which allows for the medical removal of patients in the community whose physical health is deemed to be in jeopardy. Even here, most of the cases dealt with under the legislation are older people with dementia.

Successive governments have allocated the main authority compulsorily to detain patients in hospital to the psychiatric profession. Other professions, such as social work and psychiatric nursing, take an important but secondary role. The emergence of therapeutic law in the mental health field has not been a one-way process. The struggle by psychiatry to become the dominant profession has been traditionally legitimised by its inclusion as the main profession charged with the implementation of mental health legislation for the last 150 years (see Chapters 3 and 4).

The social control function is also evident in the additional non-medical occupations, which have a right lawfully to intervene when a mental health problem is suspected. For example, police officers have only informal powers to act if someone is physically ill; but under Section 136 of the 1983 Mental Health Act they are authorised to detain for up to 72 hours, and refer for psychiatric assessment, anyone found in a public place who appears to them to be mentally ill.

The legislative mandate delegated by government within therapeutic law also has a peculiar impact on relationships between occupational groups. For example, the authority of the police to identify whom psychiatrists will see for assessment, threatens the traditional discretionary gatekeeping powers of the latter (Rogers, 1993). Thus, the existence of therapeutic law means that the state has delegated much stronger regulatory powers to mental health workers compared to other groups in the NHS. This, of course, is double-edged. Although the decisions of mental health professionals are *constrained* by specific legislation, the same law empowers them to intrude upon the lives of citizens in ways which would lead to other health workers being guilty of assault and false imprisonment. Mental health workers can lawfully intrude on resistant bodies and detain people without trial. In this sense they operate in an unusual way within the NHS. In other work contexts, such as social services, the social control function (e.g., in relation to child protection) is a common organisational norm.

The limits to professional autonomy: the case of self-regulation

A description of the various occupations within the mental health field emphasises differences in traditions, education, values, knowledge bases and skills. These factors are often cited as the core characteristics of the different professions. These attributes are often used to account for differences in status, occupational jurisdiction, remuneration and power over patients and other occupational groups.

Professionals claim a special mandate for their authority by referring to their educational standards, arcane skills and codes of practice. Thus, psychiatrists lead 'firms' of hospital teams on the basis of a purported set of expert traits, or their assumed expertise in co-ordinating and managing the work of others (Goldie, 1977). In other words, psychiatrists are superordinate in the division of labour because of their claimed unique knowledge. Their lengthy medical training, their incorporation of medical ethics, their clinical experience and their purported abilities to manage organisations all figure in this formula to account for medical 'leadership'. However, studies of the work practices of the different mental health occupations indicate that what distinguishes one occupational group from another is the extent to which they have been able to secure governmentally-endorsed autonomy over their work (Freidson, 1970). Thus dominance is an *outcome* of a successful bid for legitimacy. It is not an inevitable product of *a priori* claims to rational authority which are self-evidently valid.

Professional dominance also does not mean that one profession is superordinate against the wishes of others. Goldie (1974) showed how psychiatrists maintain their mandate of authority and how subordinate professions both challenge and *accommodate* that mandate. The latter resulted from, amongst other things, an acceptance of the medical model of mental illness as the only pragmatic basis from which to treat madness, a lack interest or concern to professionalise and a lack of enthusiasm about developing therapeutic skills. Neither does it mean that once a professional group has attained supremacy it will remain in that position. The picture of professional relationships painted by Goldie has changed significantly since the 1970s. Whilst it may still be the case that the psychiatric profession is superordinate over others, it has a much more tenuous pre-eminence.

Professionalisation during the 1980s and 1990s has been a central concern of both psychiatric nursing and clinical psychology. Moreover, the ethos of multi-disciplinary working and the relocation of professional relationships outside the hospital walls has resulted in much more complex inter-professional power relationships. Some now argue that medical dominance in mental health work is substantially fragmenting (Samson, 1995).

The inertia of the asylum: the case of psychiatrists

In Chapter 3 we noted that the rise of the psychiatric profession was closely linked to the establishment of the asylum system. Thus, its credibility and power was predicated on an administrative and managerial role as much as it was on the skills of diagnosing and managing mental disorder. In fact, credibility about the latter skills has always been difficult to sustain. Psychiatry has tended to be treated with some suspicion by others (including other medical practitioners) and it remained, until late into the twentieth century, marginalised and isolated from mainstream medicine. The 1959 Mental Health Act is often considered to have been the greatest reformist measure placing mental illness, and to a large extent the activities of other mental health workers, firmly under the control of psychiatrists. The emphasis on treatment produced a corresponding increase in power, influence and autonomy, and the medical profession's position became uncontested for many years. However, this acquisition of a dominant role can be seen as state-imposed. It was not something that was actively sought by the medical profession, but instead it was 'thrust upon them by the Percy Commission' (Bean, 1979).

> In their evidence to the Percy Commission, the medical profession suggested a weak form of treatment where the courts would (a) retain powers to detain patients in hospital after they had been admitted for a period greater than two years, and (b) allow the courts to hear appeals from any patient compulsorily detained. Proposals which involved a weak form of treatment were not acceptable to the Percy Commission. They had in mind a more logical and more radical system. (Bean, 1979, 28)

The role assigned to the medical profession in this crucial piece of legislation, which was largely reproduced with few modifications in the Mental Health Act 1983, cemented and reinforced the dominant role of psychiatry more generally in the mental health field. Arguably recent changes have acted to dilute power derived from a legal mandate. The weakening of the territorial base of the hospital and reorientation towards primary care and community settings have, to an extent, shifted mental health care away from detention and treatment in hospitals.

By 1982, between a fifth and a third of psychiatrists were working in a primary care setting. Much of this work centred on education, enhancing the skills of primary care workers and liaising between primary and secondary care settings (Strathdee and Williams, 1984). The multi-disciplinary ethos of CMHTs also makes it more difficult to transfer to the community the traditional lead role played by psychiatrists.

The strengthening of other mental health professionals' autonomy and claims to skills and knowledge have also been a key factor in weakening the traditional role of psychiatrists. Fernando (1992), a consultant psychiatrist and a Mental Health Act Commissioner, claimed that British psychiatrists currently feel under attack 'from a plethora of forces on several fronts'. He identifies these forces as coming from: the black community who criticise psychiatry for colluding with racist 'sectioning' practices; clinical psychologists who have attempted to take away the 'interesting' parts of psychiatric work, leaving doctors to deal with people deemed 'psychotic'; health services managers who have marginalised medical practitioners in decisions about the allocation of resources; and the public at large who are 'blaming psychiatrists for not curing the ills of society'. The response to these attacks, according to Fernando, has been for institutional psychiatry to:

> turn in on itself, going back to the traditional basics of medicine – emphasizing biological and genetic aspects of health and illness, concentrating on drug therapy (as an undeniably 'medical' form of treatment), devising more and more specialisms and refusing to address serious problems (such as racism) within its professional practices. (Fernando, 1992, 14)

Fernando goes on to note that despite some psychiatrists operating within a psycho-social framework, 'it is the bio-medical model of "mental illness" that is being pursued at most "centres of excellence"'. A retrenchment of this type has also been noted in the USA where demedicalisation and community mental health took place at an earlier point than in Britain. Light (1980) notes that the demedicalisation of community health, which has come about via the increased responsibilities of non-psychiatrists, has met with hostility from psychiatrists and a retrenchment into an organic medical model. We turn now to arguably the strongest challenge to psychiatry: the growth in professional strength of clinical psychology.

In the wake of 1948: the case of clinical psychologists

Clinical psychology is a relatively new profession. Its birth and growth have coincided with the NHS and for this reason it has closely followed the organisational contours, constraints and opportunities of the latter (Pilgrim and Treacher, 1992). Because a post-graduate qualification (which is now a doctorate) is required to practise, and its members claim a particular scientific mandate from their training, this has led to peculiar tensions arising with the psychiatric profession. At first, in the 1950s, when psychologists appeared in small numbers in the NHS, their psychometric assessment role posed no threat to medical dominance. A major problem emerged, though, when they made a bid to have autonomy about the behavioural treatment of people with neurotic conditions. This led to a prolonged conflict with psychiatry, which dissipated in the 1980s following the Trethowan Report (DHSS, 1977) about the role of psychologists in the NHS.

The 1980s also brought with it a shift in arenas of conflict. Clinical professions were now hedged around with the authority of general managers and so were less likely to fight amongst themselves. The relative scarcity of psychologists also gave them some advantage when the ethos of multi-disciplinary working began to take root within the health service. By the end of the 1980s remuneration of senior psychologists was catching up fast with their medical counterparts. Significantly perhaps, whereas clinical psychologists working in higher education are able to claim clinical scales of pay, alongside medical practitioners, this does not extend to psychiatric nurses, social workers or other professions allied to medicine.

Notwithstanding this challenge to medicine in terms of knowledge and technical skills, because clinical psychology is the only main mental health profession without a formal legal mandate, it has a peculiar vulnerability. Psychiatrists, social workers and psychiatric nurses all have designated roles to play within the prescriptions of various sections of the 1983 Mental Health Act, but psychologists do not. Also, the traditional division of labour of medicine – doctors diagnosing and prescribing and nurses implementing treatment – has allowed the doctor–nurse relationship to have continuous stability, which is independent of site. With the emergence now of Community Mental Health Teams and Centres, it is not clear what role a psychologist can adopt which is free from potential encroachment from other occupational groups. This encroachment is made more likely by the current orthodoxy within the profession of cognitive behaviour therapy. This, eclectic and methodologically-driven form of problem-solving with clients can be carried out by any professional trained in the approach. For example, it is now common for nurse practitioners to be cognitive behaviour therapists.

Thus, clinical psychology is currently in a contradictory stage of development (or decline). On the one hand, its numbers and remuneration increased significantly during the 1980s but, on the other, later arrangements of employment, particularly in the wake of the 1990 NHS and Community Care Act, make its practitioners vulnerable. Their role can be eroded by others and their employment is no longer guaranteed. The latter is a result of 'treatment packages' being offered in modalities which potentially could be produced more cheaply by other occupational groups (CMHNs or counsellors).

Breaking with the asylum tradition: the case of community mental health nurses

There has been a substantial increase in the number of CMHNs in the last 20 years. In 1985 there were 3000 CMHNs in the UK which was projected to increase to 4500 in 1990 and 7500 in 1995. However, psychiatric nursing has its roots firmly embedded in the asylum system. The gradual shift of services to community settings in recent years has had an impact on the style and content of work undertaken by psychiatric nurses. The changing nature of mental health nursing found official recognition in the setting-up of The *Mental Health Nursing Review* commissioned by the Department of Health in 1992 and headed by Tony Butterworth, Professor of Community Nursing at Manchester University. This was the first major review of mental health nursing since 1968, although the subsequent report, *Working in Partnership* (DH, 1994e), met with a lacklustre response from government representatives and the media.

The recommendations of the review constituted something of a curate's egg, as a result of efforts to accommodate disparate views and interests. (User-representatives and nurses from the old psychiatric hospitals were amongst those included on the review body.) In some ways the content of the report supported demands being promoted by the users' movement. For example, only limited support is given to District General Hospital Psychiatric Units as appropriate sites for nursing mental health crises and 24-hour crisis services were endorsed. At the same time, it suggested that greater attention needed to be given to the demands and needs of staff based in declining Victorian asylums.

In more general terms there appears to be a disjuncture between statements of policy and the practice and values of Community Mental Health Nursing on the ground. The assumption behind the investment in an expanded CMHN labour force has been that nurses should be focusing their attention on the needs of people with a serious and enduring mental illness (a euphemism generally for those diagnosed as suffering from chronic schizophrenia). The *Mental Health Nursing Review* called on nurses to prioritise their work with this group of people. Such a call is necessitated in part by the evidence that, contrary to the policy aim of targeting more chronic and severe cases, CMHNs have actually been directing increasing attention to people with minor mental health problems in primary care settings with, according to standard psychiatric criteria at least, limited effectiveness (Gournay and Brooking, 1994).

CMHNs as an organised interest group have departed significantly from their hospital colleagues as far as mental health policy is concerned. In particular, there is a desire from elements of the profession to distance themselves from the use of compulsory legislative powers. In contrast, hospital nurses have been keen to progress their role and status, increasing their powers of compulsion. An example of this was the inclusion in the 1983 Mental Health Act of a 'holding power', which allows nurses to detain voluntary patients for up to 6 hours (Section 5(4)). According to Bean (1986) this was not necessary and reflected the use of trade-union tactics to gain increased state recognition for hospital nurses' status and role. This example contrasts starkly with the failure of *community* psychiatric nurses to endorse the Royal College of Psychiatrists' proposal for Compulsory Treatment Orders (CTOs). This could have entailed nurses administering forced medication, by injection, in patients' own homes.

The failure of CMHNs' endorsement was an important factor in the proposed CTOs gaining legal status in the late 1980s. CMHNs argued that such a measure would adversely affect the nurse–patient relationship. The government introduced other legislative control measures, which did not centre directly on the administration of medication (Supervised Discharge Orders). CMHNs were reluctant participants, as indicated by this comment in an editorial in the *Nursing Times* (Vol. 91, No. 18, 3 May 1995): 'New legislation could fundamentally change the relationships between community-based mental health nurses and their clients. Unless nurses get involved in the debate now, they will be in no position to snipe from the sidelines once the legal framework is in place.'

Occupational substitution: the case of approved social workers

Social workers have had an established and variegated role in mental health, ranging from the introduction of a case-work approach in the 1950s heavily influenced by psychiatry and psychoanalysis, to the introduction of Approved Social Workers (ASWs) under the 1983 Act with specified duties and responsibilities in relation to the compulsory admission of patients to hospitals. The latter role acted to increase the significance of mental health work within social work practice, as indicated by the minimum requirement of two years' post-qualification relevant experience, and the completion of a specialist training course before becoming an ASW. Despite the increasing specialisation of mental health work within social work in recent years, it has not been immune from the threat of occupational substitution.

Competition between mental health workers is evident in relation to occupational territory. Occupational rivalry and encroachment can be found in most areas of health work. For example, in the area of childbirth there is the question over whether midwives should be allowed to act as independent practitioners, or whether doctors, who have a monopoly in this area, should direct the work and set the parameters of their practice. Often the state acts to resolve such struggles by agreeing to accept or reject the status claims of occupational groups, perhaps by agreeing to comparability with another group over pay, or changing policy.

Community care of people with mental health problems presents a current example in which two groups, social workers and CMHNs, are in competition. As mentioned above, social workers have a lengthy tradition of work in the mental health field. Community mental health nursing by comparison is a young profession, which has become established in the last two decades. Both are increasing in importance, given the emphasis on community-based, as opposed to hospital-based, care. Both groups lay claim to similar roles with a similar client group (i.e., those experiencing mental health problems outside hospital).

On the face of things, the knowledge base and interventions with clients of the two groups differ only in emphasis (Sheppard, 1990). The knowledge base of social workers draws on a psycho-social model of mental health problems and the social sciences. CMHNs tend to adopt eclectic psychiatric ideologies, with little attention being given to conceptual issues. There have been suggestions that because the two professions share similar skills, they are interchangeable. For example, Goldberg and Huxley (1980) claim that 'the community psychiatric nurse shares many skills with the social worker'. However, when longer-term contact with clients is considered, major differences do emerge:

The differences confirm, to a considerable degree, expectations arising from the examination of occupational socialisation and discourse. Social workers define their clients primarily in terms of social problems, whereas mental health case definitions received a higher profile amongst CPNs [community psychiatric nurses]. Social workers, according to main indicators – role, context and indirect work – operated in a wider community context than CPNs. Social workers acted as advocate or resource mobilizers, worked with outside agencies and professionals, and tackled more practical, emotional and relationship problems indirectly to a far greater extent than CPNs. Indeed, in terms of active use of community resources and agencies, CPN work appears to have been negligible. (Sheppard, 1990, 83)

However, it may suit policy-makers and certain other professional groupings to promote the substitution of psychiatric nursing for social work. Increasing the number of CMHNs forms a major part of the government's policy of care in the community, particularly in relation to case or care management. Nursing remains a profession with which medicine is comfortable. CMHNs might more readily fit in with their nursing colleagues in the context of primary health care teams. A tradition of accepting the medical authority of psychiatrists is more established than is the case in social work (Bean, 1979). CMHNs may also be perceived to be more likely to respond readily to mental health crises in the community than social workers (Rogers and Rassaby, 1986). As NHS employees, funding for CMHNs comes from the main mental health budget, whereas social workers are funded out of the smaller allocated resources of social services departments. Finally, but perhaps most importantly, CMHNs are distinguished from social workers by being charged with the administration of depot (long acting) injections of neuroleptics. Much of community care policy for those with long-term mental health problems still relies on continued compliance with, and uptake of, 'maintenance' doses of neuroleptics. In the final chapter, we address this issue in terms of whether or not the limited handmaiden role of nurses in administering a chemical fix is now part of the crisis over the management of madness.

The threat to professional dominance: the case of the police and mental health work

One of the oldest occupational groups to have a mandate in managing mental health problems is the police. Police involvement with mentally disordered people dates back to the founding of the police force in the early nineteenth century, and to its preceding constables (Walker and MacCabe, 1973). The police officer's role in welfare matters, such as mental health, has led some commentators to label them as 'the secret social service' (Punch, 1979). In this capacity, the police frequently act as an alternative to other mental health agencies. They may be the first port of call, before other services are involved, or a last resort, when alternative assistance is not forthcoming. Hospital-based mental health workers tend to work within the institutional boundaries of the hospital. Not all localities have crisis intervention teams and some social services either do not have a 24-hour service, or they lack sufficient staff to cover psychiatric emergencies.

Until recently, police officers have not generally been viewed as legitimate mental health workers. However, with an increasing number of revolving-door patients and a greater number of people now spending less time in hospital and greater periods of time living in the community, police officers have become front-line emergency workers. Consequently, their role as mental health workers has become more visible. The police are the only professional group who are in a viable position to work as 24-hour community mental health workers. Unlike other community-based occupational groups, the police force operates seven days a week and on every day of the year.

The role of the police in psychiatric emergencies has been accepted as appropriate by successive governments and is enshrined in mental health law. Section 136 of the Mental Health Act 1983 empowers the police to remove a person they consider to be mentally disordered and in need of immediate care and control from a public place to a place of safety. Under this legislation, a person may be detained for up to 72 hours for the purposes of being examined by a medical practitioner and interviewed by an Approved Social Worker, and to allow suitable arrangements to be made for his or her treatment or care. Despite official endorsement of this police role, increasing challenges have been made to the use of these powers. Considerable disquiet has been expressed from different sources, not least from other professional groups, about the appropriateness of the police having and using this mandate.

Criticism has included that made by the British Association of Social Workers and sections of the psychiatric profession. These groups have expressed reservations about the ability of police officers to diagnose mental disorder and to handle patients appropriately. However, research suggests that across a number of indicators the police are generally able to diagnose the presence of mental disorder accurately and make appropriate referrals successfully (Rogers, 1990; Bean *et al.*, 1991). The negative evaluation of police officers' competence in this area may emanate from concerns about the image and occupational control and autonomy of other mental health professionals rather than any proven failure of the police to manage mental disorder (Rogers, 1993).

Freidson (1970) identified three areas as being crucial to the attainment and maintenance of professional status. The requirements are that:

• knowledge and skills are viewed as unique and effective
• there is a monopoly and control over a market for service
• there is close supervision of training and qualifications

The police role challenges two of the requirements that are necessary for psychiatrists to maintain their professional legitimacy successfully. First, in possessing a legal mandate to bring referrals for assessment, the police can challenge psychiatric control over a market for services, including the right to choose who will be seen. Second, by making legally-sanctioned decisions regarding whether a person is mentally disordered, on the basis of 'lay' judgements, the police may be in a position to challenge the claim that psychiatrists' knowledge and skills are unique and effective.

Police work with mental health problems is much influenced by the context in which they operate and differs considerably from designated mental health services. The importance and influence of members of the public is more pronounced, decisions have to be made in the absence of case notes or previous histories, and there are uncertainties which stem from the lack of prior cues and control over external events and resources (Rogers, 1990).

Inter-disciplinary work in flux: the case of primary and community care

The police are not the only group in recent times to be given a more prominent role in the management of mental disorder. With the shift in the balance of mental health management away from inpatient provision, primary health care has come to occupy a more important position in relation to mental health care. Mental health professionals have made a shift, albeit a modest one, from hospital to primary health care settings. It has been estimated that in England and Wales as at 1993 more than 20 per cent of psychiatrists, 27 per cent of clinical psychologists and 22 per cent of psychiatric nurses spend some of their working time in general practice. The distribution of specialist mental health professionals is skewed, with most operating as CMHTs in larger 'training' practices (Kendrick *et al.*, 1993). Counselling services have also become widespread (Sibbald *et al.*, 1993). As will be discussed further in Chapter 8, general practitioners now have an increased role in the prevention and treatment of mental disorder and in the commissioning of mental health services.

The shifting location of mental health services has had a major impact on how professionals organise their work and the way in which they relate to patients and each other. The territorial base of the asylum or hospital has to a large extent been replaced by the need to negotiate one-to-one relationships in a domestic or community context.

In many ways, this shift can be viewed as giving patients more autonomy and power to set the agenda for relationships with professionals.
Mental health professionals are put in the position of having no automatic
right of entry to a patient's home, and professional/client interactions
no longer take place in a setting rich in colleagues. Thus, it may be
that clients have a new control over who they see, when, and in what
circumstances. Alternatively, faced with a choice between attending to
those who are less able to negotiate a mutual relationship and client
groups who are easy to engage and who are perceived as being most
rewarding to treat, mental health workers may opt to treat the latter.
Studies of community-based services show marked increases in rates
of inception to care for less severe mental health problems (Onyett,
Heppleston and Bushnell, 1994a).

Clearly this re-balancing of power in the patient/professional relationship has posed problems directly for professionals, and indirectly
for the state, in managing the activities of patients deemed to be a
threat to themselves or other people. In other ways the relocation of
community care provides new opportunities for abuse and neglect by a
minority of staff to go unchallenged, in the absence of a well-developed
system of monitoring and complaints procedures. This is particularly
the case with the burgeoning growth of independent hostels and group
homes for ex-patients, which are not subjected to official systematic
inspection. In this regard, the privatised nature of much residential
provision is in a similar position to the pre-regulated madhouses of
the eighteenth century discussed in Chapter 3.

Mental health workers have also been faced with the need to change
their working practices and the way that they interact. In particular,
work outside the hospital brought with it a philosophy of multi-disciplinary working, which had already operated, in theory at least, in
inpatient settings. The basic tenets of multi-disciplinary working are:
that each member of the mental health team has special skills to contribute
to the management of patients; that these are contributed in co-operation
and liaison with other mental health workers; and that this leads to the
establishment of corporate consensual goals in delivering a service.

To a large extent the implementation of mental health policy, such
as the aim to produce a 'seamless service' which overrides the division
between primary and secondary care, is predicated on notions of communication and effective liaison. Multi-disciplinary working supposedly
embodies these characteristics. However, just as corporate strategies
have failed in other arenas of public life (most notably at governmental
level and in NHS administration) there are a number of major

impediments to effective multi-disciplinary working. There is much anecdotal evidence, and some research, to suggest that rather than entailing mutuality and co-operation, inter-professional relations are characterised by defensiveness, lack of role clarity and conflict. Much of the conflict centres around bids for professional dominance or autonomy.

Psychiatrists are loth to give up 'clinical responsibility' for patients. Psychologists are developing a training or consultancy role, seeking high levels of remuneration, adopting medical titles ('Consultant Psychologist' and 'Dr') and accepting direct referrals from GPs. When working in Community Mental Health Teams clinical psychologists are reported to have low team role clarity and team identification but high professional identification (Onyett, Heppleston and Bushnell, 1994b). Threatened by deprofessionalisation, psychiatric nurses have been busy collecting more 'therapeutic skills', which can be viewed as a means of countering claims of uniqueness of skills made by the other main groups of mental health workers. Difficulties in ensuring multi-disciplinary co-operation and corporate goal achievement stem from the differing secondary socialisation and training of mental health workers. This was succinctly described by Murphy:

> Professionals in both health and social services are taught almost exclusively in isolation from each other. Doctors, nurses, therapists, psychologists and social workers plough their own educational furrows, their courses focused almost exclusively on their own professional contribution to the care of individual patients. They are rarely taught about service development during their basic training years, and multidisciplinary team working is supposed to come naturally after graduation and with experience . . . It is not surprising then to find that community teams, primary care teams and hospital based community outreach teams and social work teams rarely develop a good overview of the total service or appreciate its broader objectives. (Murphy, 1993, 20–1)

Onyett, Heppleston and Bushnell (1994b) point to the problem that team work poses for professionals around role and identity once they have been fully socialised into distinct professional groupings:

> The concentration of practitioners into teams places professional workers in a special dilemma. They become members of two groups: their profession and the team. As a result they may find themselves

torn between the aims of a community mental health movement that explicitly values egalitarianism, role blurring and a surrender of power to lower status workers and service users on the one hand, and a desire to hold on to traditionally, socially-valued role definitions and practices on the other. (Onyett, Heppleston and Bushnell 1994h, ?)

Thus multi-disciplinary success is a poor bet for politicians, as each occupational group isolates itself during training and seeks to encroach on the work of others thereafter. Such a set-up is hardly propitious for mutual goodwill or efficient and rational co-operation. And yet these are expected by the present (and past) government when ministers exhort practitioners in the multi-disciplinary 'team' to improve service quality or learn from the mistakes of service failures.

The problem is compounded by uni-disciplinary groupings emphasising the status, training level and accreditation of their own group as their contribution to improving service quality. A recent example of this is in relation to clinical psychologists spending much political effort in lobbying government ministers and trying to secure parliamentary time for a private member's bill to achieve statutory registration. Another example is the retention of systems such as the General Medical Council (GMC) and the UKCC, even though much user-dissatisfaction has been expressed about their effectiveness. By contrast a multi-disciplinary commitment to practice guidelines to standardise best practice and audit its outcome tends to be less supported by practitioners. As Hayes (1998) has pointed out, the traditional tribal self-interest of individual disciplines is in conflict with attempts to manage mental health services through a consensual commitment to principles of good practice shared by a multi-disciplinary group.

The workforce as a mirror of wider society: the case of gender and class

The stratification within the mental health workforce reflects the divisions in wider society, particularly in relation to gender and social class. However, in the mental health field these factors have interacted in a slightly different way from that of the mainstream health workforce. For example, the gendered nature of general nursing owes much to the dominance, historically, of male medical practitioners. Gamarnikow (1978) has suggested that the working relations between medical practitioners and nurses replicate the gendered nature of patriarchal society. The doctor assumes the role of patriarch, directing and determining the division of labour within the hospital setting. The nurse, acting as a subordinate 'handmaiden' to medical practitioners, augmented by concerns of hygiene and caring, takes on the role of wife/mother. The patient, as the passive recipient of care, is placed in the role of child.

In contrast to this picture of the division of labour in general hospitals, psychiatric nursing developed in a different manner. Historically, social class appears to have been a major factor in shaping the hierarchy of mental health occupations. In the nineteenth century it was principally working-class men who were recruited as asylum attendants for their strength and ability to restrain patients, not middle-class women, who were typical in general nursing (Carpenter, 1980). These attendants worked under the auspices of asylum doctors whose ranks (as with other branches of medicine) were filled by 'gentlemen of independent means'. The male, working-class position of the asylum attendants is reflected in the strong trade-union affiliation of this sector of nursing compared with the preference for the 'professional organisations', such as the Royal College of Nursing, which represented the interests of general nurses (Carpenter, 1980). Given that in both medicine and general nursing men have come to dominate the higher echelons of the professions, the class background of psychiatric nurses is likely to have contributed to the view from within nursing that its psychiatric branch is inferior to the general branch.

Thus the history of nursing can be seen to be different for its two branches, but both were a product of the interaction of class and gender influences. At the outset, general nursing provided an opportunity of respectable employment for the large pool of genteel labour being produced by middle-class Victorian families (Veblen, 1925). Abel-Smith (1960) noted that, 'If nursing could be made respectable, it could provide an outlet for the social conscience and frustrated energies of the Victorian spinster.' In the general hospital, the female middle-class matron displaced the lower-class male master of the poor-house, but she remained inferior in status and remuneration to the male medical superintendent.

At the turn of this century, nearly all of the male nurses were employed in asylums. The early nursing schools refused to admit them in case they might 'usurp the functions of doctors'. Female nurses posed no such threat, even though their class background was closer to that of doctors. We will return to this question of class and gender again below when discussing psychiatric nursing in some more detail.

Whilst the male/female dichotomy appears to be at its strongest in relation to nursing, there is evidence that it occurs in other occupational groups. Women on average occupy lower-status positions within the 'psy' professions. Pilgrim and Treacher (1992) note that female clinical psychologists are less likely to occupy managerial and professional leadership positions than men. Moreover, they found that male elements in the profession also lamented the greater proportion of women to men on the grounds that this implies an inferior status and induces a decline in salary levels (e.g., Crawford, 1989). The recognition of sexism and the relative invisibility of women within the upper echelons of the profession prompted the organisation of a separate Psychology of Women section within the British Psychological Society (Nicolson, 1992). Women also occupy an inferior status within psychiatry. Despite considerably more women medical graduates than men putting psychiatry as their first career choice and their overrepresentation in junior ranks, they are underrepresented at consultant level and in academic posts.

Conclusion

This chapter has outlined the type of knowledge and aspirations which have characterised the mental health professions separately and collectively. The case studies demonstrate the ways in which a shifting policy context is both an opportunity for professionals to advance their interests but also a constraint on that process. What is also apparent is that a stable, rational collaborative approach to service delivery cannot be assumed, given that individual professions spend time and energy on defending their interests and rebutting the encroachment of others. The final case study also illustrates that professions mirror the features of the wider society they partly constitute.

6

Patients and their Significant Others

Introduction

This chapter will address the constraints and opportunities for psychiatric patients and their significant others, which have emerged within mental health policy recently under the following headings:

- 'anti-psychiatry' and patients' rights
- the rise of the mental health service users' movement in Britain
- the professional response to users' views
- Old and New Labour on mental health
- the problem of need definition
- identifying the needs and interests of 'carers'

'Anti-psychiatry' and Patients' Rights

Concerns about the protection of the human rights of asylum inmates date back to the nineteenth century. But, as we noted in Chapter 3, those anxieties were essentially about the inappropriate detention of the sane and they have recurred in recent years. For example, in the 1990s television documentaries focused at times on the use of psychiatric services to detain and control sane people in Australia and the USA unjustly. In the case of the former USSR, Western psychiatrists themselves have compiled critiques of the 'misuse' of forced psychiatric detention for political ends (e.g., Bloch and Reddaway, 1977). This conception of psychiatric abuse assumes that 'normal' psychiatric practice is benign and legitimate: that it is 'non-abusive'. Within this view, coercive control in the form of detention and treatment is only deemed inappropriate for those 'falsely' diagnosed as being mentally ill. Similarly, diagnostic categories such as 'sluggish schizophrenia' are criticised for their pseudo-scientific status, but similar diagnoses in Western psychiatry are considered to be non-problematic. An example here is the diagnosis of 'pseudo-neurotic schizophrenia', a form of psychosis masquerading as neurosis, which only a trained psychiatrist can detect. Leaving these questions of the overlap between Western and the old Soviet forms of psychiatric knowledge aside, a much simpler question is begged about 'normal' psychiatry. If the detention and treatment of sane people is offensive and unacceptable, why is the same detention and treatment, but of insane people, inoffensive and acceptable?

The view that 'normal' psychiatry is acceptable and legitimate has been contested by dissident psychiatrists in the USA (Szasz, 1971; Breggin, 1993), Italy (Basaglia, 1981) and Britain (Laing, 1967; Cooper, 1968), and latterly by clinical psychologists hostile to biological psychiatry (Johnstone, 1992). The term 'anti-psychiatry' has often been used to describe this collection of dissenting professionals, although only Cooper (1968) used the term about his own work. The psychiatric service-users' movement emerged internationally at various points in time in the wake of these professional critiques dating back to the 1960s. We will look at the particular features of the British Mental Health Users' Movement later on in this chapter.

A number of common concerns emerged across these national developments which included hostility to ECT, major tranquillisers and the use of therapeutic law to detain citizens without trial. These aspects could also be found earlier in the writings of dissenting psychiatrists, along with other connecting threads such as a twin concern for individual freedom and social justice. The current *libertarian* aspect of user campaigning was also common in prior right- and left-wing critiques of psychiatry. For example, Thomas Szasz's work on the myth of mental illness (Szasz, 1961) and on the oppression of institutional psychiatry (Szasz, 1971) is commonly cited with enthusiasm by user-critics, who share little in common with his wider political ideology, which is right-wing. He is committed to the free-market principle in relation to any commodity, whether it be opiates or personal therapy.

Professional dissent within the mental health industry focused mainly on the conceptual weaknesses of psychiatric knowledge; the inadequacy of biological responses to social and existential problems; and infringements of the human rights of psychiatric patients. Given that these areas of dissent came to find favour with disaffected service users, it is not surprising that the latter recognised and respected the authority of the 'anti-psychiatrists'.

The Rise of the Mental Health Service Users' Movement in Britain

The work of Laing and of Cooper in Britain was largely ignored and occasionally dismissed indignantly by psychiatrists during the 1970s (e.g., Hamilton, 1973; Roth, 1973). One exception in this regard was Anthony Clare, who essentially expanded traditional theory and practice by conceding some of the arguments of anti-psychiatry (Clare, 1976). By and large, psychiatry carried on regardless in practice and consequently remained a target for criticism.

Moreover, after the 1960s a whole series of radical critiques of traditional authority had emerged which were separate from the established struggles of opposition between capital and labour. These struggles were centred on industrial tensions and had been bureaucratised in most Western countries via employers' organisations and conservative parties on the one side and trade unions and social democratic parties on the other. The separate opposition movements have come to be known as the new social movements, to distinguish them from the older labour movement. The new social movements are exemplified by struggles to advance the interests of marginalised and oppressed groups in modern society (e.g., the women's and black movements). In the case of animal rights, this has now even extended to other species. New social movements have been contrasted with the labour movement broadly on two grounds. First, they exist in a post-industrial context, whereas the labour movement was a product of an industrial mode of production. Second, the new social movements use different forms of political organisation and action. In Britain, as in other countries, the labour movement was bureaucratised and sought gains through trade-union negotiations and parliamentary representation.

By contrast the new movements often operate outside these bureaucratic forms or even explicitly criticise hierarchy and mandated authority: libertarianism is a strong and recurrent motif. One central feature of new social movements is the role of identity. Being black, being a woman or being disabled, for instance, often represents both a ticket of entry to the movement and an ongoing source of motivation and group solidarity. However, some members may not have that particular identity (e.g., 'allies' in the mental health service movement). Another feature of these movements is that they have no definitive or stable programme of action, or even organisational goals. They change, often in response to new contingencies. Moreover, within the same broad grouping there may be quite varied ideologies operating. Apart from politics being typically personalised within new social movements their other characteristic feature is the emphasis on direct action demonstrations, local and national lobbying, artistic events and forms of protest idiosyncratic to the particular cause.

With these general characteristics in mind, let us now look briefly at the rise of the British mental health service movement, which we discuss in more detail elsewhere (Rogers and Pilgrim, 1991). This movement was late in developing compared with the USA, Canada and the Netherlands. It eventually gained noticeable momentum by the late 1980s. For example, it took direct action to campaign against the moves by the Royal College of Psychiatrists to introduce some version of Community Treatment Order in 1987. Around the same time it lobbied the Advertising Standards Authority to remove a series of stigmatising posters produced by SANE. In 1988 the most significant demonstration of organisational capability was the parliamentary lobby of the shadow health minister. This entailed the co-ordinated efforts of 56 different users' groups nationwide. More recently (1999), when the current government issued its views about new mental health law, organisations such as Survivors Speak Out joined with other advocacy groups including MIND and the Mental After Care Association, and relatives' groups such as the National Schizophrenia Fellowship in joint critical lobbying.

The service-users' movement is variegated in a number of ways. First, different groups vary in their attitude towards psychiatric orthodoxy. Some believe in the abolition of psychiatry. Others seek to reform it and a small minority adhere to an illness framework and seek only to improve the treatment of 'sufferers'. Second, groups vary in their attitude towards 'allies'. By and large the latter are welcomed but there is also a current of opinion that they are a threat to the integrity of self-advocacy. Third, views vary about the extent to which energy should be expended on service development. Involvement in local consultation has been a demand of elements of the users' movement, which is now legitimised by government directives and guidance about user-involvement. However, some argue that involvement of this type diverts time and energy from wider campaigns.

What this last point highlights is a possible unintended consequence of government reforms which emphasise consumerism. The old Labourist form of health policy tended to be provider-dominated and empha-sised issues of equitable access and workers' rights within the NHS. The Conservative agenda until 1997 provided opportunities for new social movements struggling to advance the interests of the users of health and welfare services. What may not have been anticipated was that Conservative intentions about the rights of individual consumers (embodied in, for example, the Patient's Charter, with its telling apos-trophe) created a political space for the collectivist and anti-Tory aspirations of radical groups. At times this outcome was amplified by the building of alliances between the new managerial elite in the NHS and users' groups to usurp or challenge the traditional authority of medical elites (Thompson, 1987).

The Professional Response to Users' Views

The views of mental health service-users are potentially at odds with a professional viewpoint for two broad reasons. First, psychiatric patients are characterised, by definition, by some degree of temporary or permanent irrationality. As credibility is bound up with reason, then those deemed to have lost their reason also tend to lose their credibility in whole or part. The views of anti-psychiatrists described earlier challenged this logic by introducing the notion that conduct which lacks immediate intelligibility may, in fact, be understandable if the person's inner world and social context are explored properly. For their part, users more recently have suggested that their actions are provoked by various sources of oppression. This was captured in the title of the user-made television documentary, *We're Not Mad We're Angry*, in 1988. Both these approaches to rendering the irrational intelligible tend to cut little ice with orthodox psychiatry and with most forms of psychodynamic therapy. A second challenge for professionals in accepting users' views is that they may be (and often are) hostile to current psychiatric theory and practice.

Thus mental health professionals have had a number of difficulties in conceding the viewpoint of their patients. This is also the case with some social policy researchers and commentators as well. We have examined the ways in which the views of psychiatric patients have been resisted or ignored in some detail elsewhere (Rogers, Pilgrim and Lacey, 1993). Essentially four professional responses have been present:

(a) users' views unsupportive of professional interests are rejected;
(b) the irrationality of patients is emphasised;
(c) patients and their relatives are deemed to have the same interests and to hold the same views;
(d) patients' views are re-framed to suit those of professionals.

During the 1990s mental health service managers and some clinical professionals began to shift over the issue of the legitimacy of service-users' views. This was noticeable in a burgeoning number of short reports of local audits of mental health services, which included within them a sampling of patients' views of service satisfaction.

Notwithstanding these new concessions to 'patient power', it would be incautious to read too much into the potential that the emerging picture holds for patients' rights. It was certainly the case that during the 1980s marketisation and privatisation were important determinants of consumerism. However, as far as mental health services are concerned, consumerism had only a limited potential in favouring shifts of power and interests to service users. Allowing markets to regulate social relationships would always privilege the consumer. Consumers would opt for better forms of care, and inferior versions of care would wither from lack of demand. However, the NHS, the main supplier of the bulk of mental health services, has not been abolished in recent years, and neither has it been seriously privatised despite recurrent fears and claims of this from the left. Moreover, after 1997 government abandoned the previous emphasis upon an internal market and put forward a different version of quality control ('clinical governance': see Chapter 10). Also, the relevance of users as a central stakeholder group diminished within the discourse of government: for example, under the National Service Framework for Mental Health issued in late 1999 a standard is set for 'carers' but not for service users.

These general political cautions about consumerism failing to triumph in the NHS are reinforced by the particular position of psychiatric patients. A consumer model can only retain coherence if the supply of a service is regulated by demand from those wishing to use that service. But many psychiatric patients do not ask for what they get: it is imposed on them. Various sections of the 1983 Mental Health Act, like its legal predecessors, are utilised lawfully to impose restraints and treatments on resentful and reluctant recipients. In such circumstances, mental patients could only be construed to be consumers if being dragged off the street and force-fed was a feature of being a customer in a restaurant. Whether or not the principle of coercion in mental health law is deemed to be fair and reasonable, it is clear that no logical case can be made for calling detained patients 'consumers' or 'customers'.

Old and New Labour on Mental Health

In 1993 John Smith instigated a series of policy reviews ('forums') inside the Labour Party about a number of topics, one of which was mental health. The latter invited a wide membership which was not dominated by service-providers but included user-representatives, academic researchers and people working in the voluntary care sector. The overall impact of these adjustments to the previous labour movement trajectory which was unambiguously provider-led was that mental health policy from the labour movement began to show a greater sensitivity to the rights of service-users than was previously the case. In this regard, if user-campaigning has had an influence on Labour policy it raises some interesting conceptual questions about making a neat separation between old and new social movements.

A relevant existing example of the mixing of parliamentary and extra-parliamentary political forms was the common overlapping membership of the Campaign for Nuclear Disarmament and the Labour Party. With the collapse of Leninism in much of the East and the political diversification of the aims of Western social democratic parties beyond the demands of labour organisations, it may be that old and new social movements are being brought together rather than being separated. However, the signs from a New Labour government in the first three years of office after 1997 were that in many ways it was developing a much more restricted and authoritarian version of statism in its social policies. Our criticisms of the current Labour government in this regard are rehearsed in Chapter 12.

The Problem of Need Definition

The pragmatic imperatives of those commissioning and running services may obscure some unresolved underlying difficulties which continue to exist about defining the need for mental health services. One of these, already noted, is that some people receiving services are forced (usually lawfully) into the role. In what sense are they in need of a service? And according to whom: their treating professionals, their relatives, anxious strangers in public places? One framework that helps us to clarify this type of dilemma is that put forward by Bradshaw (1994). He makes a distinction between four types of need. The first of these is 'defined' or 'normative need', which is identified by professionals. The second is 'felt need' which is a subjective state of desire or want. This may be converted into the next category, 'expressed need'. Basically, this refers to people saying or asking for what they want from services. The fourth category which Bradshaw describes is that of 'comparative need'. This refers to identifying whose needs should be prioritised (the question of equity).

These distinctions are useful, but not because they solve unending debates about how to define need or reduce. What the distinctions do is highlight the potential tensions which exists between the four categories. They also suggest that policies designed to respond mainly to one type of need may fail to address needs defined in a different way. Let us take some examples in relation to mental health. First, returning to the example of the coerced recipient, we can see that services at present are shaped, at least in part, by decisions based upon normative rather than expressed need. If the latter completely determined service utilisation then no patient would be held formally under the Mental Health Act. Detained patients are in hospital because some other party has engineered that outcome (responded to normative need) and not because they have requested admission; they have not experienced a felt need and then expressed it as request for admission.

Another example is the finding that although patients prioritise talking-treatments when asked to identify which psychiatric interventions they prefer (Rogers, Pilgrim and Lacey, 1993), the treatments are actually biased towards chemotherapy and ECT. This example highlights that need definition also underpins styles of service practice. Moreover, it raises a consideration about need which lies outside Bradshaw's typology. If clinicians defend their right to clinical freedom about choice of treatment or their right to treat, are they expressing their own needs, under the guise of defining the needs of others? In other words, the current debates about need definition and needs assessment focus very much on a problematic category of 'them' (patients) and evade relevant questions about the needs of 'us' (non-patients). In practice, the latter group make decisions about the former group in the light of the needs of *both or either* party.

A third example is in relation to comparative need. A number of policy analyses have pointed out that unrewarding long-term service-users are often not prioritised by service-providers. The latter opt to work with more rewarding groups of patients. An example of how expressed needs and comparative needs may be met separately is the existence of private psychotherapy. Those patients with the ability to pay for this will have their expressed needs met (at least when the outcome is positive); however, private practice is *ipso facto* discriminatory on grounds of wealth. It excludes many people wanting it and so it is iniquitous.

Each of these examples shows something of the problem of naively assuming that services can be planned on the back of psychiatric epidemiology. They can of course be planned in this way but they would be built solely on normative need. Once expressed need is brought into play then a different service configuration might be implied. This is most clearly seen in the example of the 'Hearing Voices' campaigning/self-help group. This group of people would, on the basis of presenting with symptoms of auditory hallucinations, normally be diagnosed as schizophrenic, according to traditional psychiatric criteria. However, if their expressed needs arising from the experience of hearing voices were taken into consideration, then a singular response (aimed at suppressing the experience) would be inadequate. It would be replaced instead by a response including tolerance and various ways of negotiating meaning about the experience with the people involved.

Currently service commissioners are making *ad hoc* judgements based upon both types of input. A normative approach to planning a service inevitably will reflect professional interests, as it is built upon medical categories of information gathering. An approach based primarily on expressed needs is more likely to reflect user-interests. This might explain why users, who want the help required to live an ordinary life, get frustrated with providers, who tend to see need narrowly in terms of providing services and treatments for the illnesses they diagnose.

Bradshaw summarises the tension between a medical and social model of needs assessment by pointing out that:

> Needs assessment has emerged from and quickly settled into the language of priority setting, economic efficiency, cost-effectiveness and the market-orientated preoccupations of the political right . . . If we are to adapt a social definition of health, then we have to be involved in research on a much wider range of issues than merely the assessment of the prevalence of medical conditions. (Bradshaw, 1994, 55)

A tolerance of the co-existence of the two models of response to need is commonplace. At times, the implications of the two models are identical. An example here is the convergence of the two models about the cost-effectiveness of community-based service models. However, at other times the two models are clearly incompatible. The use of normative need to justify enforced hospitalisation is at odds with the expressed needs of people to retain their freedom.

The tension between a social model of need built upon the views of ordinary people and an official epidemiological approach also reflects a recent tension about which accounts about illness are to be privileged. When lay and professional accounts coincide then policy-makers can proceed with some confidence in their decisions. However, a problem undoubtedly arises when the views diverge. Another problem can arise when academic analysts, who are committed to an objectivist framework of population-level need analysis, remain reliant on medical knowledge, which may be distrusted by service-users.

An example is that of the work of Doyal and Gough (1991) in their *A Theory of Human Need*. The commitment of the authors to defining need properly, in order to justify equity, leads them to reject the implications of relativism and constructivism. These approaches (currently popular in medical sociology) emphasise the problem of objective definition: needs, like other phenomena studied, are deemed to be relative to time and place and are understood as being the product of negotiated meanings between parties with different viewpoints. By contrast, Doyal and Gough attempt a defence of the universality of needs. This leads them to identify what they consider to be objective indicators of 'basic need-satisfaction'.

When this model is applied to people with mental health problems it falls back squarely on to medical epidemiology. Doyal and Gough discuss 'mental disorder', along with 'cognitive deprivation' and 'opportunities for economic activities', under a notion of 'autonomy', which is separated from 'physical health'. Their indicator as to whether or not a society is responding to mental disorder is 'the prevalence of severe psychotic, depressive and other mental illness' (Doyal and Gough, 1991, 190). At no point do they concede conceptual problems about psychiatric knowledge or analyse the oppressive role professionals may play at times. For the time being, there appears to be an unresolved debate between social determinists such as Doyal and Gough and the relativist critiques of psychiatric knowledge, which have been associated with both 'anti-psychiatry' and the mental health service-users' movement. Both emphasise a social approach to need, but they differ

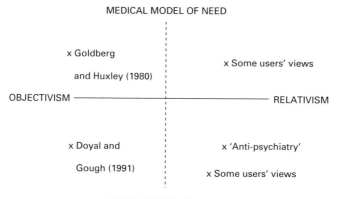

FIGURE 6.1 *Different approaches to need assessment*

along an objectivism-relativism dimension. Thus, we could situate different approaches to need assessment within four boxes produced by the intersection of two dimensions, as in Figure 6.1.

It can be seen that we have placed 'some users' views' in two places in Figure 6.1. This is to indicate that the users' movement contains a mixture of ideologies. Most of the users' movement can probably be situated in the bottom right box. The largest users' organisations, such as Survivors Speak Out and United Kingdom Advocacy Network (UKAN) are examples in this regard. They are consistently critical of medically-dominated services and they emphasise rights of citizenship. However, some are in the top right box. An example here would be that of the small users' group associated with the National Schizophrenia Fellowship (Voices). This accepts the medical label of schizophrenia, describes users as 'sufferers' and accepts the likelihood that the condition is biologically caused. However, these people also defend their right to be heard about the quality of service delivery from their own experience and perspective.

What is clear is that the top half of the diagram implies a response to need dominated by *services*. By contrast, the bottom half of the diagram implies a response to need based mainly around social rights. The right half of the diagram emphasises a lay perspective, whereas the left half emphasises the views of *experts*. These different emphases highlight and return us to a point made at the start of this section: definition of needs are contested and they reflect underlying tensions about knowledge, as well as power.

The issues of knowledge and power, and their expression through interests, is a focus of the analytical work on consumerism in the NHS by Williamson (1993). She makes the valid point that an emphasis on interests takes us further than power and knowledge alone:

> Consumerism in health care is often discussed in terms of knowledge or power, as if it were consumerism in commerce. I think that looking at consumerism in health care in terms of interests offers a more liberating analysis. It allows the dynamics of the convergences, conflicts and interchanges between consumerism and professionalism to be understood with sympathy towards both sides. It recognises that although some people lack power or knowledge, they always have interests and that when their interests are met, they do not need to secure them through knowledge or power. It takes account of the existential and not merely the political weakness of patients. (Williamson, 1993, 2–3)

Williamson extends the work of Alford (1975) about structural interests in health care (see Chapter 1) in order to unpack the ways in which the interests of professionals and those of patients can be antagonistic or complementary. Her two main dimensions of analysis are synergistic/non-synergistic interests and dominant/repressed interests (see Figure 6.2). Synergistic interests are compatible or concordant ones.

For example, for our purposes we might think of the depressed patient successfully seeking help from a psychotherapist or a GP prescribing anti-depressants. In this case the interests of the patients (to be helped) and those of the professionals (to be paid a salary and deploy a treatment they like) are both being met. However, at other times interests may be incompatible or discordant. An example here might be the person who is depressed and reluctantly agrees to ECT. The person feels under duress but is too low to protest and goes through a frightening and unhelpful experience. The professional prescriber of ECT, on the other hand, has his or her interest met (by using a treatment of his or her choice).

The other concept Williamson (1993) uses is that of dominant interests. This is a rephrasing of the established work on medical dominance within medical sociology (Freidson, 1970; Turner, 1990). Basically, clinical professionals – especially, but not only, medical practitioners – have interests which prevail over patients. There are clearly degrees of this. The surgeon faced with patients who for crucial periods of time are unconscious has more opportunity to exert his or her domi-

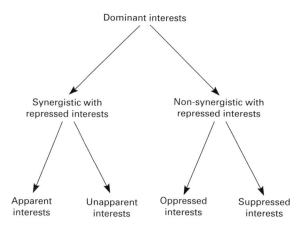

FIGURE 6.2   *Synergies and non-synergies between dominant and repressed interests*

Source: Williamson (1993).

nance (both before and during operations) than a GP who relies on building a long-term, voluntary and compliant relationship with patients. In the case of psychiatry, too, a range of contingencies may arise along this dimension. When therapeutic law is used to detain or treat patients against their wishes then it is clear that their interests are being repressed. By contrast, patients who work out a treatment plan with their psychiatrist do not have their interests repressed.

To complicate matters Williamson also notes that people are not always aware of their interests being met or denied. Figure 6.2 outlines her view of the four different outcomes in practice when the dominant interests of professionals are either synergistic or non-synergistic with repressed interests. Applying this set of outcomes to mental health we could envisage the following examples.

1   *Apparent interests*: A CPN carefully checks with patients' morale and asks whether they require any extra home visits. The patients are fully aware of this activity, are grateful for the professional's consideration and happily accept the invitation for more contact.
2   *Unapparent interests*: A social worker spends an hour ringing various housing agencies to find a placement for a patient awaiting discharge from a secure hospital. The patient is not aware of this activity.

3 *Oppressed interests*: A service-users' group campaigns without success to have a leaflet it has produced on the hazards of psychotropic medication made available to all patients in a local DGH psychiatric unit. The users are fully aware of what is happening but, for the time being at least, professional power has blocked their demands.

4 *Suppressed interests*: A patient new to the psychiatric system is given major tranquillisers but not told anything about the iatrogenic risks involved in their use. Here staff withhold important information, which keeps the patient in ignorance and jeopardises that person's health and well-being.

The strength of Williamson's analysis lies in it going beyond a simplistic conceptual and political opposition between consumerism and professionalism. These two aspects *are* opposed at times but at other times they are not. Without a framework for examining the ways in which the interests of users and professionals may in various ways either coincide or clash, one is left having to be either pro- or anti-professional. Williamson's framework for this reason has a sophisticated explanatory potential. For example, to return to the range of user-group views we mentioned above, it is rare to find users who believe that psychiatry should be abolished (the Campaign for the Abolition of Psychiatry, CAPO, has but a handful of members in Britain). Equally, the National Schizophrenia Fellowship users' group, which adheres conventionally to a medical model of illness, is a minority position within the users' movement as a whole. This framework also contains the possibility of a convergence of the collective interests of users and professionals.

Having reviewed the issue of needs and then reframed it as one of interests, it becomes apparent that the meeting of various needs and interests can be analysed as a *dynamic* between groups of social actors (in our case mental health workers and service users in the main). The problem with limiting the discussion to needs alone is that it is always vulnerable to the problem of individualism. Needs ultimately are defined and explained in terms of states inside individuals, who are always patients or clients and very rarely professionals. Clearly these needs do exist: people are distressed and some of them want and may obtain help. But the states are only part of a wider picture in which interests are also in play *between* groups of individuals. The collective interests of these groups can be analysed separately from individual needs.

Identifying the Needs and Interests of 'Carers'

Throughout this chapter we have discussed users' needs, interests and demands. Informal carers have also been identified as an important interest group in both the provision and the burden that caring imposes, mainly on women (Finch and Groves, 1980). There is a particularly large body of literature about the provision of forms of community care by the family which entails tending and nursing tasks. However, informal care in the area of mental health is not the same as that associated with carers of people with physical illness or disabilities or of children or elderly people. The distinctions that have been used by social scientists to analyse the carer's role (i.e., the distinction between caring for and caring about) are not altogether transferable to mental health. More than any other group of carers, the relatives of people with mental health problems, particularly those diagnosed as schizophrenic, have been implicated in the identified patients' symptom presentation. This is not only true of the arguably sexist view put forward by 'anti-psychiatrists' (Laing and Esterson, 1964) that schizophrenia is primarily related to the 'double-binds' that mothers impose on their children, but also of more mainstream research which illustrates the importance of expressed emotion in 'relapse rates'.

The relationships between psychiatric patients and their relatives are complex (Pilgrim and Rogers, 1999a). Situations may arise in which relatives may care about a person but at the same time be very distressed or frightened by their actions. A person who will not get out of bed or acts in a chaotic and menacing way is clearly not easy to live with and will undoubtedly upset his or her relatives. Whether the strain and distress the latter experience and are expected to tolerate constitutes caring for the identified patient is a moot point. As Perring, Twigg and Atkin (1990) point out, the most important question in this regard is 'What is it like to live with someone who is diagnosed as mentally ill?' Psychiatric patients may at times need others to tend to their physical needs but more frequently need others to tolerate, adapt to or cope with their oddity. The latter can be both distressing and disruptive to family life. In consequence, relatives of people with mental health problems often develop psychological distress of their own. Indeed, relatives express the need for psychological support and clear information from statutory services in this coping role (Goldberg *et al.*, 1993).

Given this complexity about the notion of informal care in mental health, the needs of relatives should have separate consideration within mental health policy and provision. It may not be assumed that their needs and difficulties are the same as those of the carers of other groups of people, nor may it be assumed that their needs are the same as those they care for.

Whilst the simple distinction between being a carer and being a disabled person is ambiguous in relation to physical disability (e.g., disabled women may care for their children and/or vice versa), it is even more complex in the case of people with mental health problems. A psychiatric patient may live at home and care for either children or older relatives. Also, the relatives of psychiatric patients may be angry and resentful about the intimate contact which is imposed on them because they share the same household. Relatives feel obliged to care for the person with problems in their midst. However, intense domestic relationships may then aggravate the mental health of both parties. But sometimes the reverse will apply, and family support will be enabling to people with mental health problems, as, for example, in patients returning to the community from secure facilities (Norris, 1984).

A final peculiarity of the carers' role in relation to mental health problems is at the collective level. Whereas carers' groups in the area of physical disability are usually marginal or powerless in relation to social policy, this has not been the case in relation to mental health policy. Groups dominated by the interests of relatives such as the National Schizophrenia Fellowship and SANE have often engaged in high profile campaigns which have overshadowed the public profile of patient-centred groups such as MIND (Manthorpe, 1994).

Notwithstanding this complexity of roles, research on the impact of community-care mental health reforms in Italy on female relatives living with psychiatric patients reported results which indicated surprisingly low levels of 'burden'. The findings of this research suggest that economic prosperity and employment opportunities for women outside the home may act as important social support mechanisms in cushioning the negative aspects of living with someone with a severe and enduring mental health problem (Samele, 1993).

Conclusion

During the 1980s, the sources of consumerism as an ideology were linked narrowly to the New Right agenda about shaping public services in the image of businesses in a market-place. However, this process had unintended consequences. It spurred or reinforced the growth of a new social movement of disaffected service-users. In turn, the latter challenged the worker orientation of the labour movement in relation to health policy, as well as traditional medical elites. At present a Labour government in power appears to be more concerned about supporting the interests of the relatives of psychiatric patients rather than service-users themselves.

7

From Mental Illness to Mental Health?

Introduction

Most of what are called mental health services actually respond to people with a diagnosis of mental illness. In this chapter, we consider the issues of mental health promotion and prevention in its broader social context. As institutions recede not only as a means of incarceration but also from the public eye, influences on mental health and well-being from within broader social life take on greater salience. This includes the social and personal factors that make people vulnerable to mental distress, and aspects of the environment that promote or inhibit psychological well-being. It includes the way in which the public, government and community agencies include or exclude those with mental health problems and accept or reject them as 'citizens'.

Prevention has traditionally not been a central plank of mental health policy. However, there are signs that this trend is changing. Mental health prevention and promotion are assuming an increasing salience in policy-making alongside other social policy reforms designed to promote social inclusion. Mental health promotion and prevention now form an explicit part of a wider government strategy for addressing inequalities in mental health status and access to resources and services (DH, 1997). They constitute a significant strand of work carried out by the late Health Education Authority in England and its Scottish equivalent (The Health Education Board for Scotland). However, this renewed commitment to tackling mental health inequalities exists in tension with other policy priorities which are embedded in the expanding public and political concerns about the perceived risk attached to community mental health provision. Thus policies which rely on increased coercion sit uneasily and militate against those designed to enhance citizenship.

The Marginal Place of Prevention and Promotion in Mental Health Policy

Primary health care and preventative medicine were central assumptions which underpinned the establishment of the NHS. The anticipated effectiveness of this branch of the new health service led some of its advocates to predict optimistically that the health service would constitute a diminishing drain on public funds, as it reduced and prevented illness. However, the dominant resource position assumed by the hospital sector meant that acute services were prioritised over primary and preventative services. This imbalance has never been rectified (Berridge, Webster and Walt, 1993). However, the trend in favour of the secondary care sector began to be reversed in the 1980s, when primary and preventive services were given greater priority within resource allocation and planning of the NHS. More recently, health promotion has been widely pursued as a policy goal. This can be seen as a reaction against the prevailing bias in the orientation and structure of the NHS towards curative medicine. It also reflects an increasing recognition of the importance of the cultural recognition of the role of environmental and 'risk' factors, dietary habits and stressful living in the generation of illness.

Whilst health promotion and prevention overall have had only a limited place in health policy, this trend is even more pronounced in the area of mental health. Traditionally the focus of health promotion policy has been predominantly on preventing physical ill health. This is reflected in the WHO strategy of 'Health for All' by the year 2000 which, despite a holistic approach, gives a low priority to mental health within its statement on prevention. It included only one mental health goal from the 38 identified: the reduction of the suicide rate (Thornicroft and Strathdee, 1991). This priority was transported into the most recent public health document, *Our Healthier Nation* (DH, 1998). The reason for the marginal status of mental health within health promotion strategies is in part related to the way in which services have been structured and mental and physical deviance dealt with historically. Both mental health and preventative medicine were a focus of nineteenth-century government reforms. Different strategies were adopted to deal with each of these. As we have seen in Chapter 3, the way in which Victorian society dealt with emotional deviance was by mass segregation in asylums. The threat of moral contagion posed by mental illness was dealt with by removing it from the sphere of civil society and community. A separate set of sanitary reforms constituted the basis of attempts to deal with the threat of infectious disease.

Thus despite policies and action emerging over a similar time span, a clear demarcation between physical and mental health took place and the two policy topics became *administratively* separate. Similarly, more recently, government policy in the area of mental health has focused almost exclusively on community care, hospital run-down and de institutionalisation, whilst health promotion strategies have emphasised the social causes and potential prevention of physical ill health. Questions about mental health have generally focused on organisational arrangements, not on environmental or lifestyle factors. An exception to this low policy priority about the promotion of mental health is the strategy adopted by the government in the immediate aftermath of the Second World War. As with many policy areas, war seems to focus government action in a way which eludes routinised peacetime policy-making. As we have seen, the period within and around the Second World War was significant in introducing mainstream service provision, therapeutic communities and psychological treatments. Similarly, the government instituted Civil Resettlement Units (CRUs) to provide for ex-prisoners of war. As Newton (1988) points out:

> Although the evidence as to their effectiveness is lacking they were clearly intended to be a preventative service. After three or four weeks with their family, the ex-prisoners of war were offered a stay of a few weeks or months at a nearby CRU. The centres provided an opportunity to rest and recuperate, to learn about post-war civil life, to get specialist advice and to rediscover their previous work skills or acquire new skills. The average stay was about five weeks and ex-prisoners were assisted in their efforts to reintegrate into the civilian community and especially their home environment. They were given vocational guidance and help in finding work. Furthermore, their families were offered advice on how best to respond towards and support their returning kin. (Newton, 1988, 13)

Newton's phrase 'clearly intended to be preventative' signals a connotation of the latter word which lay people would rarely use. It refers to the reduction of existing impairment or the chance of relapse (see discussion on tertiary prevention below).

A number of other barriers to placing preventative practice at the centre of the mental health work are also evident. First, *conceptual vagueness* has been an impediment to the planning of preventative services, research and policies. The wide-ranging notions of prevention (primary, secondary and tertiary) mean that the concept covers everything from vulnerability factors and macro-social problems to the providing of treatment and care to prevent recurring crises. A wide range of definitions has been deployed in policy which relate to a range of individual factors and implicate a variety of interactive processes between individual and environment.

Second, *research has had a lack of influence* on practice, policy and the delivery of services. Whilst there is still a dearth of research and evaluation on the effectiveness of social and economic policy initiatives, there are examples of conditions where the impact of interventions is marked, which strongly implicate a certain type of service provision but which have not been implemented on a wide scale. The separateness of the organisation of research and clinical services is likely to be an important factor (i.e., the university versus the 'clinic'). Policy-makers are on the whole influenced by practitioners, who have the main responsibility for setting up and running projects. As Newton notes, 'Public policy has tended to be influenced more by enthusiasm than evaluated information and information has been generalised to problems it was never meant to solve' (Newton, 1988, 10).

Third, despite the drawing-up of long-term plans of service delivery, until recently planning has been characterised by *ad hoc-ism* and incrementalism (i.e., making minor adjustments to existing arrangements). Planners are anxious to be seen to be 'doing something'. In contrast, re-orientating towards prevention requires extensive changes to existing arrangements and personnel, and the results of prevention policies are often difficult to measure. Managers and commissioners of services are under pressure to demonstrate a short-term impact of their decisions, but mental health promotion/prevention may not fit well with this.

The seemingly clearer agenda of physical compared to mental health has frequently meant a downgrading of mental health promotion programmes even in the absence of evidence or evaluation of the efficacy of such programmes (Macdonald and O' Hara, 1998). Also, as we explore below, prevention implicates social variables and processes which have until recently fallen outside the jurisdiction and potential control of health services. The introduction of a public health approach to health promotion discussed below is a deliberate attempt by government to reverse this trend.

Finally, there is also a problem related to the focus of clinicians. They have a vested interest in the identification and treatment of disorders rather than prevention. The latter requires different approaches and personnel. The leap from being a medical practitioner to a housing and employment 'broker' is a big one. Additionally, as we noted in Chapter 5, 'generic' working and an increased focus on community-based prevention clashes with a tradition of separate mental health professions and the socialisation and treatment emphasis of mental health practitioners which militate against such role flexibility.

Notions and Concepts of Illness Prevention and Health Promotion

The arena of health promotion and prevention is highly contested. Terminology is rapidly changing and signifies competing positions and orientations.

1 The *medical model* of health education and prevention is the most established and traditional approach. This focuses on bringing about attitudinal and behavioural changes in individuals. This individualistic emphasis is augmented by population-level interventions, such as mass vaccination against infectious diseases.

2 The *educational model* is drawn from a more voluntaristic model in which information transfer encourages individuals to opt for more healthy habits. It is the style and orientation of these first two approaches that differs rather than their substantive content.

3 Criticism that these two approaches are too focused on individual behaviour, or 'victim blaming', has led some to try to shift the agenda to more socially orientated models of health promotion or a *'new' public health* model. This approach emphasises environmental, social and economic conditions and seeks to transcend the traditional boundaries of public policy (e.g., housing, health, transport). In seeking to improve the health status of individuals and communities it includes both health education and all attempts to produce environmental and legislative change conducive to good public health; it also places a priority on wider questions of social policy which can alter these factors. This approach incorporates the activities of lay populations in setting agendas for health and necessarily adopts an eclectic strategy to improving health, combining education, information, community development, local citizen participation, health advocacy and legislation.

Those who initially advocated this position were influenced by The Black Report on inequalities in health published in 1980 which had focused on the materialist causes of health inequalities (DHSS, 1980).

This approach has had variable success. At a local level, community initiatives, which involve 'healthy alliances', started to emerge and a health promotion approach has been reinforced at an international level by the World Health Organisation (WHO, 1985) who initiated a 'Health for All' campaign, as an attempt to shift from a narrow medical approach to health prevention. However, notwithstanding these successes, until recently this approach has had a modest impact. The 1980s were not conducive to tackling the root cause of inequalities. The lack of recognition of the importance of community and society more generally was evident in the change of terminology used to differentiate health disadvantage (from 'health inequalities' to 'variations').

The interests of central power are often incompatible with a focus on the mobilisation of community groups and on the material causes of ill health (Little, 1990). The late 1990s saw a resurgence of interest in inequalities in health and greater receptivity to this at the level of government. An independent inquiry into reporting of health inequalities at the end of 1998 made a number of recommendations which implicated reducing income inequalities, improved opportunities for work and availability of social housing (HMSO, 1998). We discuss in the penultimate section how the tables have recently turned back towards such an agenda in the UK.

Mental Health Promotion versus Prevention

It was seen earlier that there has been a variety of approaches to health promotion and prevention. A distinction between health promotion and illness prevention is also evident in the mental health field. A mental illness prevention approach has a narrow focus (Tudor, 1991). It derives from the natural sciences and, in particular, medicine. Also, it has been located in the institutions of public health/welfare, at a particular historical time and place in the development of the welfare state. In other words, an emphasis on illness will inevitably tie prevention to the knowledge base, practices and institutional forms of a single profession: medicine. By contrast, mental health promotion is informed by a different set of assumptions, which underpin positive attempts to create or preserve mental *health*. This entails an inherently political strategy, which targets social and material aspects of society. It is also an approach which envisages the involvement of other groups of people apart from medical professionals:

Community mental health promotion is that work done to promote the positive mental health and well being of individuals, groups and communities, whether geographical or organisational work carried out by a range of professionals involved in the field of mental health and of health promotion as well as by members of that particular community – and mental health and well being as defined by those individuals, groups and communities. (Tudor, 1991)

The focus of British mental health policy has *not* to date been influenced by this broader tradition of health promotion. For this reason, what we report below mainly focuses on mental illness prevention strategies. Disease prevention has been classified by its medical advocates as primary, secondary or tertiary in type. *Primary prevention* refers to steps taken to anticipate and pre-empt disease occurrence. *Secondary prevention* entails intervening at an early stage in disease causation and/or occurrence. *Tertiary prevention* is concerned with minimising the effects associated with existing illness and so refers to the prevention of relapse or the minimisation of subsequent impairment. For this reason, in practice it overlaps substantially with treatment. In psychiatry, treatment is often cited as having a prevention or relapse function.

This threefold categorisation is more appropriate when applied to physical ill health, where the chain of causal events and factors are generally (though not always) easier to define than in the case of mental illness. None the less, it provides a useful framework to analyse the policy and practice surrounding mental illness prevention.

Primary Prevention

The United States: a case study

In contrast to Britain, where there has not been a discernible primary prevention policy, North America has a history of such a focus. In the USA, the 1960s saw the emergence of a movement which believed that mental health problems could be prevented through wide-ranging changes to the social structure. This radical primary prevention ethos was rooted in two traditions: the community mental health movement (CMHM) and psychiatric epidemiology. The CMHM emerged at the time of reforms which introduced community mental health centres in the USA. This was designed as the main plank of a policy to shift the locus of care from state hospitals to the community. A national network of 2000 CMHCs based on local catchment areas was set up.

The remit of the CMHCs was not only to provide alternatives to hospital care but to have a public health focus in preventing mental illness and promoting mental health. This philosophy was informed by a view that the cause of mental health problems could be located in society and social problems. Put another way, social structures and processes, rather than the individual, were deemed to be 'psychotoxic'. Accordingly, CMHC staff were to view themselves not only as clinicians but also as social activists.

If the reduction in the incidence of mental health problems is taken as an indicator of the success of primary prevention strategies, then the CMHM failed in its aspiration. This failure has been attributed to a variety of factors. Some argued that the commitment to a prevention strategy was hampered by the persistence of a medical model within mental health services. Certainly there was wide-scale opposition to this part of the CMHC's role from those adhering to a more conventional psychiatric position. Social activism was dismissed as a 'flight from the patient' (Dunham, 1967) and as a 'psychiatric band-wagon' (Burrows, 1969). There were other reasons for why innovative projects failed. In particular, there was a lack of clarity about the relationship of social factors and processes to mental illness and a simplistic notion of power in the community, which was deemed to be 'the therapeutic dyad writ large' (Wagenfeld, 1983).

This lack of focus had its roots in the knowledge base which provided the impetus and ideology for the CMHM. Community studies conducted in the 1950s and 1960s (Hollingshead and Redlich, 1958; Myers and Bean, 1968) suggested links between social conditions and disadvantage (e.g., unemployment, poverty and racism) and psychiatric morbidity. Whilst these studies were able to say something significant about prevalence rates (e.g., that rates of schizophrenia were far higher in 'lower' social classes than higher ones), there was a lack of data on the incidence of mental disorder. This meant that the linking factors between cause and effect were not established. In fact, because causal pathways were never properly identified, few clues were provided as to where interventions could be most effectively targeted. The studies were also criticised for being overly social in failing to consider the contribution of endogenous (genetic) and other individual factors (Weissman and Klerman, 1978).

Despite the failure of this first primary prevention strategy, a second generation of US preventive initiatives has been identified (Wagenfeld,

1983). Whilst not forming the impetus of a new social movement (see Chapter 6) in the way that the first did, it was based on more clearly focused processes and objectives. The Task Force set up under the Carter administration to examine mental health differed in two major respects from the CMHCs' approach: first, a hierarchy of scope and specificity of interventions was identified; second, there was a recognition that preventative strategies, with their focus on the social, lay outside the remit and values of mental health professionals.

The underlying knowledge base emphasised a different level of analysis from that of the community studies discussed above. The approach was influenced by social epidemiology, which viewed the onset of mental distress as being linked to changes in life events and the social world of individuals (Dohrenwend and Dohrenwend, 1974). In other words, the emphasis shifted towards *precipitating* rather than predisposing factors and consequently sought to reduce the prevalence of mental health problems, but not necessarily their incidence. Prevalence refers to the aggregate number of cases recorded in a population at a point in time, or new plus old cases. Incidence refers only to recorded new cases. A model of prevention which seeks to identify and remove primary causes to reduce incidence is clearly more ambitious than one which seeks to lessen the stress on vulnerable individuals to reduce prevalence. Thus, preventing mental illness now focused on eliminating stressors or minimising their deleterious effects. The type of interventions implied by this model ranged from strengthening social networks to brief crisis counselling at the time of a threatening life event.

It has been pointed out that a shortcoming of this approach is that it ignores the social factors emphasised by the first generation of primary prevention, namely ageism, racism, sexism and classism. It seems that one of the major problems of primary prevention is that the level of analysis, where prevention is deemed to be crucial, excludes important factors operating at other levels.

A third conceptual framework for primary prevention is one which focuses on stages in the life cycle (i.e., stressors pertinent to infancy, early childhood adolescence, adulthood and elderly people). Targets for intervention involve socially, psychologically and biologically induced stressors: for example, the deleterious behavioural consequences of toxic psychoactive drugs on the central nervous system for all ages are such legitimate targets. For older people, preventative goals might involve the maintenance of cardiovascular, renal and pulmonary function as a means of retarding the onset of psychological symptoms; alteration of living arrangements to reduce the noxious effects of sensory deprivation; or targeted interventions to reduce the enormously increased risk of morbidity and mortality associated with widowhood (Wagenfeld, 1983, 174). Wagenfeld views this approach as complementing and strengthening the precipitating life event model of prevention, as it has the capacity to include biological factors.

It is interesting to consider why a strong tradition of primary prevention emerged in the USA and not elsewhere. In Britain, there have been attempts to establish a prevention of mental illness agenda but these have not had a major impact on mental health policy formation. Three important factors appear to be the differences in Britain compared to the USA, and these concern: the radical politics of the 1960s; the community care focus of mental health policy-makers; and the nature of psychiatry.

The timing of community care initiatives began earlier in the USA than elsewhere. The libertarian *Zeitgeist* of the 1960s entailed so-called 'anti-psychiatry' emerging in several countries (the USA, Britain, France, Italy) in different forms. However, the fact that de-institutionalisation occurred earlier in the USA than elsewhere is likely to have been an important factor. In Britain there was a politicisation of mental health but this mainly lay in a radicalisation of the therapeutic community movement. Consequently, in the USA, it was understandable that radical mental health workers turned their attention to reversing what in the community seemed to be responsible for the creation of mental health problems.

A further factor in the USA related to the presence of a segment of psychiatry which was dedicated to social epidemiology. This tried to uncover the social roots of mental health problems. Social psychiatry has a tradition in Britain too, but this has tended to focus on the production of secondary deviance generated by large mental hospitals (Barton, 1959), and secondary or tertiary prevention, as in the work on expressed emotion discussed in more detail below.

The Secondary Prevention Emphasis in Britain

GPs and primary health care services have been targeted as agencies for the secondary prevention of mental health problems. The rationale for this is that GPs are the officially designated gatekeepers of health services, and the first port of call for patients. Because of their ready accessibility, GPs are likely to have contact with most of their patients on an annual basis. Goldberg and Huxley (1980) suggested that over a period of a year, over 90 per cent of patients deemed to be suffering from a mental disorder made contact with their GP.

A focus of those advocating a concerted approach to secondary prevention is the screening and diagnosis of mental disorders. It has been estimated that through everyday consultations 'family practitioners are able to detect 60 per cent of all mental disorders'. However, formal screening devices are considered to yield higher detection rates (Falloon and Fadden, 1993). Mental distress is considered to be frequently masked by somatisation (the presentation of physical signs and symptoms) which may make detection more difficult. The use of formal diagnostic tools, such as the Present State Examination and Mini Mental State Suicide Risk schedule, are thought to increase detection rates, thereby allowing earlier intervention and referral to services.

However, different stakeholders hold differing views about the value of GPs accurately identifying the presence of psychopathology. Psychiatrists, who have been the main proponents of screening and who have been instrumental in the design of tools specifically for this purpose, tend to view early screening as a self-evidently desirable goal. Moreover, they see GPs being guided in this task by the psychiatric profession. For example, Creed and Marks (1989) state: 'Support and advice from psychiatrists enables GPs to improve their care of patients with psychiatric and psychological problems.' As a result of this input, the authors go on to say, 'the skills of general practitioners and their trainees are enhanced'. There has been a less enthusiastic response from some GPs who view the relationship between GPs and psychiatrists as an unequal and increasingly irrelevant one as GPs form new relationships with workers in other mental health disciplines such as psychology, counselling and social work (Ferguson and Varnam, 1994).

There is also evidence that users might not always place the same value on the screening and detection of mental illness as psychiatrists do. The fact that GPs are sometimes poor diagnosticians, as judged by traditional psychiatric standards, and hold views closer to lay definitions of mental health problems means that users may *prefer* them to specialists. Moreover, it is interesting to note the discrepancy between the traditional psychiatric views outlined above about the tendency of GPs to miss mental health problems through somatisation, and the views of users in the same study who claimed that at times GPs fail to take seriously their physical complaints.

Reducing the suicide rate: a flawed secondary prevention strategy?

There has been increasing focus within government policy on the high and growing levels of suicide in society. Epidemiological and other research reflects a dramatic increase in the rates of suicide. The suicide rate amongst young men has doubled over the last two decades and accounts for approximately 2000 deaths a year amongst people aged 15–35 in England and Wales (Office for National Statistics, 1997). Official concern with suicide was expressed in *The Health of the Nation* (DH, 1992b) which identified primary health care workers, and GPs in particular, as key agents in reducing the suicide rate. More recent public health policy, which takes a more multi-sectoral approach (as expressed in *Our Healthier Nation*, DH, 1998), also identified a reduction in the suicide rate as one of its main targets in improving the mental health of the population.

Whilst government targets have shown improvement overall the scope for reducing the suicide rate is limited, given the present strategy. Official policy implicitly assumes that suicide is a direct manifestation of mental illness. The rationale then goes like this: psychiatric morbidity needs to be detected and treated, and this early intervention will reduce the incidence of suicide. However, both the range of assumed causes and the official categorisations of suicide are complex. The risk of suicide in relation to most mental disorders *is* high. Estimates of risk suggest between a fivefold and fifteenfold increase (Harris and Barraclough, 1997). Nevertheless mental illness may not always be an antecedent correlate, let alone a 'cause' of suicide. There are many people who commit suicide whom any psychiatrist would not label as mentally ill (e.g., those with a terminal illness or those who, for existential reasons, consider their life to be over).

Even for those who have had a previous history of mental illness, their psychiatric condition may not be the main precipitating factor. High suicide rates amongst psychiatric patients have been associated with social factors such as living alone and substance misuse, as well as 'clinical factors' (Appleby *et al.*, 1999a). Context and access to lethal substances are also likely to be implicated. For example, pharmacists have one of the highest rates of suicide because of their access to the effective means of taking their own lives. Similarly, many of the psychoactive drugs given to mental health service users, if taken in overdose, are lethal. Hence, it may be ready access to large amounts of toxic drugs which is primarily implicated in the suicide of some social groups such as pharmacists and psychiatric patients. In the latter

case, psychological disturbance may be compounded by medical prescribing norms in relation to anti-depressants, major tranquillisers,
anti-Parkinsonian agents and other drugs. If polypharmacy (more than
one drug being prescribed at the same time) is present, then both intended
and unintended self-harm increase in probability

There are other possibilities too. Paradoxically, the detection and
treatment of a major mental illness may actually contribute to the suicide
rate. The pessimism surrounding the diagnosis of schizophrenia, the
iatrogenic impact of major tranquillisers, regular compulsory detention,
and being unemployed and unemployable, might cumulatively lead to
a *rational* appraisal in patients that their lives are not worth living. In
other words, psychiatric patients are not just diagnosed as being ill:
they are subjected or exposed, in that role, to a series of events which
create depression and anomie. Indeed, many psychiatric patients diagnosed
as schizophrenic, who are living in the community, struggle not with
active symptoms of psychosis but with the apathy and demoralisation
arising from their social marginalisation (Barham and Hayward, 1991).

In *The Health of the Nation* targets were criticised for paying 'little
attention to tackling the social conditions associated with this problem' (Baughan, 1993). The strategy emphasised screening and changing
individual behaviour, whilst ignoring the structural influences implicated in suicide. Baughan points out the importance of negative life
events, particularly attitudes towards and experience of unemployment
in youth suicide. This analysis implies the need to reduce youth unemployment and improve social conditions more generally. In addition,
greater consideration may need to be given to the provision of counselling services in further and higher education rather than in GPs'
surgeries. The cultural norms of machismo may make it less easy for
young men to admit to emotional problems either to informal networks
or more formal counselling services. Thus, anti-sexist education in
schools, together with education in dealing with personal troubles in
the school curriculum, might be an effective way of raising awareness
of dealing with intractable life situations and stressful life events (death,
unemployment, divorce, etc.). It might also reduce the stigma of 'help-
seeking' amongst young men.

Labelling is also likely to play a significant role in who is, and who
is not, defined as a suicide risk. The recognition and labelling of the
act of suicide varies socially and culturally and is affected by the categorisations of a multiplicity of agencies, including medical practitioners,
coroners and those who collate official statistics. One particular consideration is who is likely to be labelled as a 'suicide risk'. For example,

are depressed young white women more likely to be viewed as a risk than young black men diagnosed as schizophrenic? Does the latter diagnosis discourage professionals from formulating the problems of psychotic patients in personal and social terms? How are *attempts* at suicide viewed by health service personnel, whether genuine attempts, cries for help or manipulative gestures? All of these relevant factors are not addressed by a blinkered effort at diagnostic screening. Moreover, will a reliance on the traditional secondary prevention skills in primary care and directing interventions purely at the symptoms of mental illness be effective in the longer term?

Tertiary Prevention

Whereas the hallmark of secondary prevention is accurate initial screening, tertiary prevention has a different focus. It is geared towards minimising the impact of mental illnesses on patients' lives and preventing the 'relapse' of recurring disorders such as 'schizophrenia'. The purpose of screening by mental health professionals here is to identify, and if possible intervene in, the determinants of psychopathology, in order to minimise the probability of distress recurring. Interventions are generally pitched at the level of the individuals or their family. Most of these strategies are aimed adjusting the individuals to their social context.

There have been a number of important research findings in recent years which has suggested various ways of minimising the recurrence of disorders. These are mainly psycho-social interventions. The identification of biological vulnerability is limited. However, acute episodes of mental distress are linked at times to nutritional variables, the effects of physical disorders, brain damage and the effect of drugs (Falloon and Fadden, 1993).

In the area of those with a diagnosis of schizophrenia, the work of Brown and his colleagues implies certain policy strategies to minimise the recurrence of acute mental distress. From this work two sets of findings about the social environment of vulnerable people suggest ways of reducing the prevalence of acute episodes and improving the quality of life of patients. A study carried out by Brown and Wing (1962) indicated that understimulation and total institutional settings were found to result in withdrawal and regression. On the other hand, overstimulation was found to be detrimental too. Brown *et al.* (1966) noted that patients discharged to a hostel rather than back into a family setting often did better. Exploring this observation further, in subsequent studies, people with a diagnosis of schizophrenia are more likely to relapse where they are discharged to families expressing 'high expressed emotion' (a combination of critical comments, hostility and 'overinvolvement'). Family therapy and educational models aimed at exploring family dynamics and reducing levels of expressed emotion have also been found to be successful.

Cross cultural studies have also pointed to preventative strategies. In India, where long-term recovery rates are better, studies suggest that families with a member who has been labelled as schizophrenic are far less likely to show evidence of high expressed emotion than in Britain. A further observation implicating the broader social and economic environment has also been made by Warner. A study of the political economy of schizophrenia (Warner, 1985) suggests that developing countries are more conducive to recovery than Western nations. Developing countries appear to promote greater reintegration and the rehabilitation of social roles for people who have had a psychotic breakdown. This more successful resocialisation seems to be linked to a combination of family patterns of support, with low levels of expressed emotion; a return to valued work roles; and a lower level of stigma about mental illness. In the West, ex-patients often end up unemployed or confined to doing menial low-status jobs in occupational schemes with poor pay. A further indication that the social context rather than individual factors is important is the longitudinal study in Europe by Ciompi (1984), which has shown that social opportunities for worthwhile employment are a much better predictor of recovery than severity of diagnosis.

From the above discussion, it is clear that the social environment of people diagnosed as schizophrenic is a central feature in tertiary preventive policies. The reduction of expressed emotion in the family, the provision of adequate and suitable non-family-based accommodation and employment opportunities, and a flexible and tailored mental health management plan which involves the patient's family, are all implicated. And yet there is little evidence that such approaches are widely adopted in contemporary psychiatric practice. There remains a reliance on large doses of major tranquillisers, coupled with the belief that 'schizophrenics' do poorly in response to psychological treatments. Thus there appears to be a major gap between the psychiatric literature on what is known about tertiary preventative practice and its actual implementation.

The rise of a public health approach to mental health promotion and inequalities

Most of the secondary and tertiary definitions about mental health are reliant on the illness model and as we have seen they have focused on secondary and tertiary strategies. In recent years there have been attempts to shift towards adopting more positive notions of mental health which are distanced from these more medicalised definitions. This is evident in the Health Education Authority's (HEA) definition: 'Mental health . . . is the emotional resilience which enables us to enjoy life and to survive pain disappointment and sadness. It is a positive sense of well-being and an underlying belief in our own and others dignity and worth' (HEA, 1996).

Elements of mental health have also been viewed as a part of a set of increasing or decreasing psycho-social elements (Macdonald and O'Hara, 1998): environmental quality versus deprivation; self-esteem versus emotional abuse; emotional processing versus emotional negligence; self-management skills versus stress; social participation versus social exclusion. Within this reframing of mental health there has been a growing emphasis on how lay people understand and construct the notion. Recent studies show that lay people tend to adopt a relative, rather than an absolute, view of mental health which focuses on the interplay between material circumstances and psychological well-being (Rogers and Pilgrim, 1997). However, a difference from more formal definitions is that it seems that people expect negative emotions to be part of everyday life, and separating the negative from the positive aspects of mental health does not relate easily to everyday experience (Pavis, Masters and Cunningham-Burley, 1996).

The association between socio-economic status and mental disorder has been clearly established and recognised for many years (Henderson, Thornicroft and Glover, 1998). More recently, theorising within health inequalities has tied emotional and psychological health more closely to theorising about inequalities more generally. Importance has been attributed to the notion of social capital which refers to 'features of social life-networks, mores and trust that enable participants to act together more effectively to pursue shared objectives' (Putnam, cited in Wilkinson, 1996, 221). This notion implies that the quality of social relationships and, most importantly, our perception of where we are relative to others in the social structure, are likely to be important psycho-social mediators in the cause of inequalities in health.

These changes in the discourse about mental health have been attended by the emergence of a broader 'public health' approach to mental health promotion, which encapsulates the growing emphases on holistic and social definitions of positive mental health. The Green Paper, *Our Healthier Nation: A Contract for Health 1998*, constituted the centre-piece of the incoming Labour Government's agenda about public health and for tackling health inequalities more generally. A broad and inte-grated approach which extends well beyond the individualist focus of its predecessor, *The Health of the Nation*, is evident in the notion of a 'contract for health' and the idea that connected problems which ema-nate from multiple influences operating at different levels require a 'joined up approach' to their resolution. These two notions encompass an acknowledgement of the relationships between individuals (micro level), organisations (meso level) and government (macro).

This integrated comprehensive approach means that interventions are not aimed solely at the individual (micro level) but also focus on the structural conditions and processes at the meso and macro levels and interdependence between these levels. Mental health promotion has become part of this broader public health focus. Since 1997 there has been a significant increase in area-based initiatives aimed at regenerat-ing deprived communities and reducing poverty and social exclusion. Health Action Zones (HAZs) incorporate aspects of this new approach to public health. They have been sent up to link health, urban regen-eration, employment, education and housing initiatives to respond to the needs of vulnerable groups and deprived communities. As arche-typal complex community-based initiatives they have three defining characteristics (Judge, 2000). They aim to:

(a) promote positive change in individual, family and community circumstances;
(b) develop mechanisms to improve socio-economic, physical circum-stances services and conditions in disadvantaged communities;
(c) place an emphasis on community and neighbourhood empowerment.

Intra-urban patterns have been a prominent and enduring feature of ecological studies of mental health which have shown the highest rates of admissions in inner-city areas (Henderson *et al.*, 1997). Thus, a key change in the focus of the new public health approach, which has been to consider the impact of neighbourhoods and localities on people's health, has particular salience for the promotion of mental health.

Whether or not this approach is more successful than the primary prevention approach in the USA discussed above awaits the outcome of evaluation, which itself forms an intricate part of the development of the new approach. However, some questions are begged. First, will the absence of a range of mental health outcomes hinder the focus on mental health in a more general strategy designed to reduce health inequalities? The identification of suicide rates as a proxy measure for mental health is very limited but remains the key target for mental health outcome in *Our Healthier Nation*. Second, will this broad sweep approach enable full participation in social and economic life and be able to deal specifically enough with the social exclusion experienced by those with a mental health problem? Third, will a swing to a concern with risk and safety undermine attempts made to redress social inclusion and exclude people with mental health problems further? Whilst the government seemingly subscribed to an ethos of listening to users, its emphasis on the so-called threat posed by those with a mental health problem suggests this may not create a conducive climate in which the needs and experiences of people with mental health problems are attended to. Despite the pursuance of an official policy of social inclusion things might turn out differently, as Judge (2000, 37) suggests: 'we need to recognise there there could be a very different future in store – one in which social exclusion becomes ever more pronounced for some groups and individuals, and ever more inescapable for people with a diagnosis of serious mental illness'.

Conclusion

This chapter has reviewed a set of debates about mental health promotion and the prevention of mental illness. It is clear that, until relatively recently, neither of these has been high on the agenda of the mental health policy formation process in Britain. We noted earlier that prevention has not been a priority in British mental health policy. Examples of primary prevention strategies have come from the USA and have had little impact here. Our secondary prevention strategies have proved modest in their remit and implementation in practice. Tertiary prevention is something that is widely discussed by social psychiatrists in Britain but there is little evidence of it being put into regular practice. We discussed the possible reasons for the emergence in the USA of a strong primary prevention tradition and its absence in the UK in the context of the politics of mental health during the 1960s.

A refocusing on positive notions of mental health and a re-emergence of debates about mental health have added to a new public health model which holds out considerable potential in relation to improving mental health in populations and reducing inequalities. The extent to which this new approach is successful in part will depend on a multiplicity of ways in which the social exclusion of those with mental health problems are dealt with in services and in the wider community. The mass de institutionalisation of psychiatric patients threatens to undermine a policy which ostensibly seeks to redress inequalities and promote social inclusion. Thus the way in which we treat those with mental health problems as citizens in a wider sense is important. We return to this theme at different points in our remaining chapters.

8

Primary Care

Introduction

In the past, primary health care has been favoured by central government as the site for the secondary prevention of mental health problems. (In the last chapter we noted that secondary prevention entails early screeening and 'nipping problems in the bud'.) The rationale for this is that GPs are the designated gatekeepers of health services, and the first port of call for patients. Because of their ready accessibility, GPs are likely to have contact with most of their patients on an annual basis. Goldberg and Huxley (1980) suggested that over a period of a year, over 90 per cent of patients considered to be suffering from a mental health problem made contact with their GP. Recent estimates suggest that between 10.5 and 13.5 per cent of those considered to have severe and enduring mental health problems are managed at the primary care level (Callanan *et al.*, 1997).

This chapter is concerned with exploring the rising profile of primary care within mental health policy and practice. With de-institutionalisation, primary care has shifted from simply being a 'filter' or referral pathway to the secondary care sector to being a site of specialist activity. It is also the main site for the management of people with a range of mental health problems living in the community. This has been reinforced by a series of government-led changes over the last 10 years which have significantly altered the role of primary care. Prior to de-institutionalisation, primary care staff had a relatively marginal role in the management of mental health problems. Latterly, primary care has become a sector which provides the main source of official management of people with depression. It employs a mental health work force of its own and is now in a position to commission and run services which previously lay outside its remit. All these changes have meant adjustments in the way in which primary care has conceptualised itself and how other parts of the health and social care sector respond. It has also fed into wider trends such as the expansion and legitimation of counselling and talking therapies.

Definitions of primary care

Primary care has been defined in a number of ways. It has been conceptualised as the utilisation of the various sources of care available to respond to new illness episodes and as a social concept concerned with populations as well as individuals. This includes the less visible self- and informal primary care provided by non-professionals (Ashton and Seymour 1988; Rogers and Elliott, 1997). A more traditional definition entails primary care being constituted by the organisational aspects of formal service provision, such as general practice and primary health care teams, with other practitioners operating at the periphery. Elements of the latter definition will be the main focus of this chapter, although the former, wider definition has considerable relevance to the final section when discussing the relationship between formal primary care and the wider community.

General Practitioners and Mental Health Care

GPs are being expected increasingly to fulfil both a secondary prevention and an aftercare role (which subsumes tertiary prevention). For some time after the setting-up of the NHS, GPs operated in the shadows of their hospital counterparts and so they attempted to emulate hospital medical practice: 'The recurrent concern about trivial demands, the desire for hospital work, and the emphasis on academically acceptable foundations are all examples of the continuing influence exerted by the consultants over their generalist colleagues during this period' (Calnan and Gabe, 1991, 145). This relationship of general practice to mainstream hospital provision was embedded in the legislative and other arrangements pertaining to mental patients during the 1950s and 1960s. A clear reflection of this subordination to specialists is the role designated for GPs in the assessment of patients for compulsory admission to hospital. Compulsory admissions under the 1983 (and previously the 1959) Mental Health Act generally require two medical recommendations, one from a psychiatrist and the other from a registered medical practitioner with personal knowledge of the patient. The GP fitted the latter role. The thinking behind this combination was that each of the medical practitioners could bring something different to the assessment: the psychiatrist his or her specialist knowledge, and the GP his or her personal knowledge of the patient.

In theory, the idea envisaged by the designers of the mental health legislation specifying medical recommendations (under the 1959 Act) was that the GP could act as a corrective to the psychiatrist's assessment, if the need arose. In practice, however, GPs probably rarely challenged the authority of psychiatrists who, as the 'specialists', were likely to be the key decision-makers (Bean, 1986). Comparisons of GPs' and psychiatrists' decision-making indicate that GPs' decisions are strongly influenced by the presence of a previously acquired psychiatric label in making referrals, whereas there was no similar influence on psychiatrists in their decisions (Farmer and Griffiths, 1992). This suggests that in relation to mental health legislation and referral, GPs have traditionally viewed themselves as subordinate to their hospital colleagues. (Of course, things may change under new mental health legislation in which legal and lay parties may acquire a greater say in matters compared with treating psychiatrists or other medical practitioners than has traditionally been the case.)

In relation to diagnosis and the ability to detect and manage mental disorder, specialists too have traditionally viewed GPs as inferior psychiatrists. Moreover, appropriateness of referral and treatment are largely defined and operationalised by psychiatry. GPs' skills and capacities have been viewed in a way which is commensurate with their role as 'generalists' rather than 'specialists', and therefore as having limited legitimacy in managing mental health problems.

This view may have been reinforced further by the way in which GPs have been identified in the wider community with problems in relation to the prescribing of benzodiazepines (minor tranquillisers). During the 1970s and 1980s these drugs, which were widely prescribed by GPs, came to be associated with addictive and dependency-inducing properties. Young or middle-aged women suffering from anxiety and depression were portrayed in the media as the victims of inadequate care by GPs (Bury and Gabe, 1990). Litigation and vociferous campaigning from addicted campaigners and cautions from professional bodies, such as the Royal College of Psychiatrists, led to the number of prescriptions of these drugs falling by a third during the 1980s (Medawar, 1992). The gap to a large extent has been filled by an expansion in counselling in primary care and by alternatives such as beta-blockers and newer anti-depressants such as Prozac (this is the tradename of a drug produced by Eli Lilley which acts on the neurotransmitter, sertotonin). Prozac and similar agents have been presented by the media as miracle drugs. GPs prescribe them for a range of conditions, such as panic attacks, generalised anxiety, eating disorders, and obsessive-compulsive disorders (Lyon, 1996). There are, none the less, continuing doubts about the legitimacy of the GP as a prescriber of powerful psychotropic drugs. Part of this view, at least on the part of people seeking help from mental health services, seems to stem from the concentration of GP attention on the prescribing of drugs to the exclusion of identifying and managing the social and existential problems which lead people to contact primary care services in the first place (Rogers and May, forthcoming).

Notwithstanding the questioned legitimacy of GPs in relation to selected mental health matters, there are suggestions of a more complex relationship emerging between primary and secondary care professionals. Outside the operation of mental health law, secondary care professionals may have less of an influence over GP action than has previously been thought. There are indications that a proportion of GPs view their link with psychiatrists as increasingly irrelevant as new relationships develop with workers in other mental health disciplines such as clinical psychology, counselling and social work (Ferguson and Varnam, 1994). Additionally, the findings of a systematic review of research into the impact on primary health care providers of attaching mental health professionals to their teams suggest that the latter have a limited, short-term effect on practice workload and costs. While patients are under the care of mental health professionals, doctors' consultation, prescribing and referral rates are lowered. However, the changes are modest and do not appear to be sustained in the long term beyond 6 months (Bower and Sibbald, 1999).

The pattern and nature of mental health provision in primary care has changed significantly in the last 15 years. This can be seen as resulting from two interlinked influences. The first, which we have discussed extensively throughout this book, concerns the changes outside primary care which have brought about a need to provide for the medical requirements of patients residing in the community, rather than in hospital. The second set of factors are related to the organisational and ideological changes within primary care which have altered the ability of those in that sector to have a greater influence over the shape of and provision of mental health services.

Tensions at the Interface between Primary and Secondary Care

Traditional primary and secondary care arrangements between specialist and generalist medical practitioners were disrupted by the introduction of CMHTs. These increasingly became the main referral point through which GPs and other primary care sources gained access to the secondary sector. This arrangement replaced that of GPs referring to psychiatrists.

There have also been raised expectations that primary care workers would become participants in the Care Programme Approach (CPA: see Chapters 9 and 12). A shift in focus by the secondary care sector to concentrate on the management of those with a long and enduring mental health problem meant that a large number of patients (e.g., those diagnosed with depression) previously referred from the primary care to the secondary care sector were now expected to be dealt with exclusively within primary care. Policies designed to shift care from hospital to primary care have been accompanied by moves to persuade primary care to adopt models of shared care as a means of improving the relationship between primary and secondary care. The intention was to provide a 'balanced' and 'seamless' service between the primary and secondary care sectors. Four models of care have been identified which are broadly designed to support primary mental health care (Gask, Sibbald and Creed, 1997):

(a) *Community Mental Health Teams* – these provide increased liaison and crisis intervention;
(b) *the 'shifted outpatient clinic'* – psychiatrists operate clinics within health centres;
(c) *attached mental health workers* – (usually) CPNs are designated to work with those with mental health problems in a primary care setting;
(d) *the consultation-liaison model* – this provides primary care teams with advice and skills.

However, these have not always proved to be popular options within primary care and have not been widely implemented to date. In relation to the attached mental health professional model there has been increasing pressure for CMHNs to be withdrawn to work with those considered to have a severe and enduring mental illness. This, together with the unacceptability of a solution not directly under control of primary care professionals at a time when they were rapidly gaining the power to direct services autonomously, is likely to have been an important factor in the non-proliferation of the attached worker model. The consultant-liaison model, which has not generally been considered to have been effective in resolving disputes about referral criteria or changing GP behaviour, has operated with the assumptions of the secondary care sector (e.g., reducing rather than increasing referrals of minor mental health problems; enhancing GP skills in the detection of mental health problems). Whilst advocates of these models argued that they would provide improvements in community care and bring primary and secondary services closer together, from a different standpoint the proposed solutions can also be viewed as a strategy of those in the hospital specialist sector to retain traditional control over an area which was being encroached upon by primary care.

The Organisational Power to Influence Mental Health Developments within Primary Care

There has, over the last 30 years, been a significant organisational shift of practices from single-handed to group practices. Primary health care teams, which include nurses and health visitors, with GPs employing clerical and other staff, have been well established for a number of years. These organisational changes provided GPs with the opportunity to employ staff such as primary care counsellors directly and for primary care nurses to become more directly and explicitly involved in mental health. There has also been a shift in the knowledge base of GPs towards a biographical approach. This has created an easily identifiable knowledge base which marks general practice off from other medical specialties. This approach stresses the need to engage with patients in a holistic manner and to view their illness in the framework of their biography and social circumstances (Armstrong, 1979). These changes have also been important in terms of incorporating mental health fully within the ambit of primary health care in so far as they have built on innovative minority practices already in operation. For example, the Tavistock Clinic pioneered the attachment of social workers and others in primary care, and the group-case seminar approach of Balint (1957). Commensurate with this is the more recent 'patient centred' approach to managing patients' problems which has also grown and influenced ways of working significantly within general practice (Stewart *et al.*, 1995). This approach places an emphasis on the psychological and social needs of patients as well as medical needs by identifying a number of defined professional values. These include finding common ground (with the patient) regarding management, incorporating prevention and health promotion, and enhancing the patient–doctor relationship.

Radical changes in the structure and organisation of services over a number of years have provided the foundations for transforming mental health care in primary care. The lack of a history of specialist knowledge about mental health and the administrative expectations from central government about such issues as involvement in care and case management, supervision registers and referral to CMHTs has been countered by the ability of GPs and their managing authorities to control developments more from within the terrain of primary care. The creation of Family Health Services Authorities (FHSAs) in place of Family Practitioner Committees in 1990 fortified the provisions for directing the activities of GPs. The FHSAs brought with them the power to allocate funds for new developments. Mental health was one of the developments to benefit from such funding, and some FHSAs created the opportunity to fund independent mental health workers directly to work in primary health care (Goldberg *et al.*, 1993). The balance of power shifted further under changes brought about by the NHS and Community Care Act 1990. Many GPs became budget-holders and purchasers as well as providers of services up until 1997.

In the mid-1990s, total purchasing and fund-holding arrangements permitted a general practice or groups of practices to hold delegated budgets with which to purchase secondary care services for their patients. Thirteen sites around the country also operated as mental health extended fund-holding pilots between 1996 and 1998 with the ability to purchase inpatient mental health. Closer and more effective working relationships between primary and secondary care were effectively stimulated by these projects (although there was little impact on relationships with social services). However, as with the models of interface working described above, there was also evidence of conflicts at times over the priority that professionals working within the different sectors had about the criteria of need when setting the agenda about mental health priorities operating in different localities. The primary care fund-holding sites were more interested in providing primary care-based services to a wide constituency whilst professionals working in the secondary care sector were more concerned to concentrate specialist mental health services on those designated as the 'seriously mentally ill' (Lee and Gask, 1997). The advantage of these pilot sites for general practice was that innovations in practice provided new models of mental health working which distinctively bore the hallmark of primary care. However, the disadvantage of these arrangements was that because total fund-holding arrangements were not always tied into locality-specific developments in mental health this created a tendency towards anarchy, with fund-holders failing to conform to local mental health strategies.

The wish to abolish the internal market relationship between 'pur-chaser' and 'provider' formed the backdrop to the proposals set out in the Government White Paper, *The New NHS: Modern and Dependable* (DH, 1997). Primary Care Groups and Trusts (PCGs/PCTs) are currently being established in England, Wales and Scotland. These new bodies, which have responsibility for commissioning all primary care services with an integrated independent budget, heralded a major change in the provision and commissioning of health and community care services. The explicit aim of setting up PCGs and PCTs was to attune service provision to local needs by improving the quality, range and accessibility of services, tackling unmet need and developing organisational models of health care delivery which could integrate community with primary care.

In the mental health field these developments have brought with them opportunities for service innovation which were not possible (or were problematic) under the old arrangements. Larger commissioning and provider groups created a wider and different range of services, making it easier (in theory) to provide a planned and comprehensive primary care counselling service than has been possible for GPs or health centres working alone. The obligation of these new entities to develop partnership working also raises the possibility of primary care service developments which involve users and build relationships with a range of voluntary community groups concerned with responding to the everyday social and material needs of people with mental problems.

Early evaluations of PCG activity present a mixed picture in relation to these aspirations. There are suggestions that whilst mental health is recognised as constituting an important priority for improving the health of the population for a significant minority of PCGs, service development horizons are limited only to the expansion of counselling. In one study carried out in 1999 by the National Primary Care Research Centre, a majority of PCGs reported no intentions to develop general practice-based mental health services. Moreover, it is clear that mental health is seen as a priority for developing (specialist) community services much more than as a priority for general practice-based provision. Few PCGs are taking the lead in commissioning specialist mental health services, with most reporting that they have no direct involvement in commissioning.

The Rise and Rise of Primary Care Counselling?

The growth in counselling has been the major signifier of an expanded primary care mental health agenda. Counselling services are widespread in general practice (Sibbald *et al.*, 1993). Recent estimates suggest that over half of all practices in PCG areas have on-site primary care counselling. Despite the popularity of establishing counselling services in general practice which is, in part, reflected in the positive evaluations that patients provide about talking therapies, there are also questions about its efficacy. In the 1990s counselling services grew rapidly and without regulation, raising questions about the quality and effectiveness of service provision which have yet to be resolved (Sibbald *et al.*, 1996). The findings of a randomised controlled trial of the comparative cost-effectiveness of counselling, cognitive behaviour therapy and usual GP care in the management of depression suggest that counselling may hasten recovery but, in the longer term, there are no significant differences in health gain or costs of care.

Primary care counselling places GPs in a strong position to purchase the type of mental health services they think most fits their patients' needs. Thus, GPs may decide to buy psychological services direct from clinical psychologists or employ counsellors on a sessional basis in their surgeries. As well as the effectiveness of counselling other issues are relevant to address which relate the the quality of care provided within primary care. Primary care counselling is unlikely to meet the diversity of mental health needs in primary care. Whilst it may prove to be a 'quick' fix for GPs in terms of providing a readily accessible disposal route for those with psycho-social needs it may not meet more complex needs. The need for a variety of types of support to resolve problems and the use of new models of care together with other more traditional options are currently at risk of being excluded.

Primary Care as Part of a Wider Mental Health System

Limits to the new-found freedom to direct services more closely from within the terrain of primary care are constrained by external expectations about quality enhancement. This coincides with a more general move on the part of central government agencies to specify the nature and content of service provision, rather than the broad generalised aims with few expectations which characterised policy-making prior to the mid-1980s. *The National Service Framework for Mental Health* (NSF) published in 1999 (see Chapter 12) identified primary care groups as the lead organisations for access to mental health services. Standard two of the framework states that any service-users who contact their primary health care team with a common mental health problem should 'have their mental health needs, identified and assessed and be offered effective treatments including referral to specialist services for further assessment, treatment and care if they require it'.

The assumptions about the responsibilities in relation to promoting access to services in Standard three are onerous, particularly as they include the need for primary care organisations to act as facilitators and co-ordinators of other agencies. This is stipulated in the NSF as residing not only with general practice but with local health and social care communities who need to establish explicit and consistent arrangements for access to services around the clock:

- via the GP or primary care team
- through NHS Direct and other help lines
- in Accident and Emergency (A&E) departments through mental health liaison services with a gateway to specialist services through effective out-of-hours arrangements
- via access to services for people detained by the police.
- through making information readily available for people with mental health problems, including access to self-help groups and support services such as housing and employment.

Evidence will need to be provided that services respond to mental health needs quickly, effectively and consistently 24 hours a day, 365 days a year.

The relationship between where responsibility for successful implementation, and its failure, lies is not clear, although the PCG is identified as the lead organisation. Performance will be assessed nationally in terms of improvements in mental health outcomes. These include a long-term improvement in the psychological health of the population, as measured by:

- the National Psychiatric Morbidity Survey
- a reduction in the suicide rate
- the extent to which the prescribing of anti-depressants, anti-psychotics and benzodiazepines conforms to clinical guidelines
- access to psychological therapies

- the experience of service-users and carers, including those from the black and ethnic minority communities.

In addition to the specific standards relating to primary care and access, primary care groups and general practice are identified as being key partners in the other six standards. The biggest challenge faced by this centrally-directed framework will be in providing the necessary capacity to deliver what is set out in the NSF. The baseline working assumption of the NSF acknowledges the lack of this capacity within primary care, and accepts that local health and social care communities need to enable primary care to manage common mental health problems and to refer for specialist advice, assessment and care appropriately. On other fronts it will be a test of new partnership workings (e.g., the extent to which PCGs can ensure lay involvement and extend their remit to other agencies such as criminal justice agencies). Ensuring access requires a focus on, and an ability to influence, secondary care arrangements. Working with health authorities and local trusts will be essential in order for this to happen. Primary care providers will need to deal more directly with issues of public safety. This emphasis within current mental health services has been outside the routine concerns of GPs whose tradition is largely about voluntary relationships with their patient group.

Implementation of the NSF at the level of primary care provision is likely to involve major changes in roles and responsibilities in relation to mental health. Primary care has gained experience of commissioning mental health services, which has acted to reinforce existing interest among some GPs. However, this has been very much a local bottom-up initiative and there is also evidence to suggest that a considerable number of GPs remain ambivalent about, or indifferent to, mental health matters.

The Changing Relationship between Primary Care and Public Health

The emergence of the NSF, together with other changes outlined in this chapter, suggest that the focus of primary mental health care provision is beginning to shift as both general health and mental health policy is being resited and reconceptualised. A counterbalance to the disproportionate concentration on the relationship between primary and secondary care are attempts to refocus primary care outwards to respond to mental health need in local communities. The Green Paper, *Our Healthier Nation* outlined an approach which places an onus on primary care workers and other local health agencies in developing strategies that can respond to both the local sources of distress and their impact on patients and potential patients. Whilst a substantial amount of mental health need finds its way into primary care, there is also evidence of a considerable 'iceberg' of unmet need in which mental health problems go undetected. For example, a study of women's pathways to primary care for post-natal depression found that 80 per cent had not reported their symptoms to any health professional (Whitton, Warner and Appleby, 1996).

The potential of primary care to impact on mental health at the level of populations rather than individuals is evident in the latent function offered by primary care in areas of deprivation. For example, an evaluation of a nurse-led primary care service in Salford illuminated the way in which local people viewed the practice as a perceived source of stable social and emotional support. This could be reliably accessed in the face of an increasingly disruptive environment which had resulted in the erosion of sources of social support and networks (Chapple *et al.*, 2000). The ambitions of the NSF standards in primary mental health care discussed above are, to a large extent, reliant on primary care developing access and services at the interface between primary care and local communities and populations. Both a general and more specific mental health focus to align a public health approach to mental health problems is discernable in recent policy developments. Community-orientated primary care (COP) is an attempt to place primary care more firmly at the centre of health care and to fuse it with the concerns of a social vision of public health. COP has been defined as:

> the continual process by which primary health care teams provide care to a defined community on the basis of its assessed health needs by the planned integration of public health with primary care practice . . . It stands in a long tradition of attempts to fuse the practice of community medicine and primary medical care. (Gillam and Miller, 1997)

However, to date, formal attempts to engender a 'public health focus' in relation to mental health have proved elusive. In an evaluation of COP it was found that mental health was easily marginalised in setting an agenda for action in the schemes, as intimated here by Gillam and Miller (1997, 29): 'although in most teams there was a desire to tackle mental health problems (stress, misery, loneliness, the effects of unemployment), such topics were usually rejected. Reasons included a lack of control over the causes and the absence of effective interventions'.

Within general COP schemes, where mental health competes with other areas of interest, the primary care team, as well as individual GPs, may simply fail to move beyond the shortcomings of an individualised and medicalised approach to mental health work. Where mental health development is prioritised from the start over other issues, a public health focus may be more successful. The principal preconditions for development in this area have been identified as including: a strong user-orientation; clear 'project champions'; a holistic service development approach; culturally appropriate provision; a non-hierarchical team structure; an assertive approach to community development; an enabling balance between statutory and non-statutory sectors; and long lead-in times to development (Callanan *et al.*, 1997).

Conclusion

Primary care has become a major force in mental health policy over the last 20 years. Yet its passage has not been smooth or established with ease. The mental health problems with which primary care was associated were framed increasingly in mental health policy debates as 'minor' and were gradually excluded from the ambit of new community and secondary care services. The latter were increasingly targeted at 'the seriously mentally ill'. This nomenclature often misleadingly implies that 'minor' equals 'less distressing'. The term 'serious' tends to allude consistently to social dysfunction or disruption; it does not always mean 'seriously distressed'. Thus the discourse of 'minor', 'moderate' and 'serious' remains highly problematic but the marginalisation of primary care at times has been a function of the notion of serious mental illness being seen *ipso facto* as more important in policy developments.

The development of mental health care within primary care over this period may be viewed as attempting to increase the legitimacy of both general practice and the status of mental health problems, such as depression and anxiety. Primary care involvement in mental health formed part of the struggle to extricate general practice from its subordinate position to secondary care. In reality this meant general practice promoting itself as a distinctive and competent profession to deal with mental health in the face of criticism about the GPs as inferior mental health workers. During the 1980s primary health care workers, and GPs in particular, were vulnerable to a number of accusations about their potential lack of success as (part-time) mental health workers. They were faced with legitimation problems about the prescribing of minor tranquillisers and having to work in subordinate ways to the secondary care agenda at a time when general practice was attempting to reverse its subordination to hospital medicine and assert its independence, embedded in an original knowledge base and arena of practice.

The National Service Framework now places a substantial onus on primary care to improve mental health provision. Whether it succeeds will depend on new commitments from GPs about mental health as an issue and on the ability of specialists to shift into, rather than trying to control, primary care working. We also note in this chapter that the service horizons of primary care will need to be raised beyond that of simply enlarging the availability of counselling.

9

Community Mental Health Care

Introduction

As we noted in Chapters 3 and 4, mental health care over the last two centuries has been dominated by the rise and fall of the asylum. Moving from institutional to community settings has triggered a whole new mental health enterprise called 'community care' or 'care in the community'. In some ways, the idea of community care in mental health ran counter to the dominant trend within the NHS after 1948, which, until recently, was centralised and hospital-dominated. Latterly, 'community care' has been an emotive term within a policy context. It has tended to draw venom and passion in equal amounts from both policy-makers and commentators. On the positive side community care has held out the promise of a humanitarian solution to oppressive institutions. On the negative side, 'the community' has been seen as a dustbin into which all but the most dramatically dangerous, and hence politically embarrassing for society, problems can be dropped. Such strong contrary views have been influential in both driving and retarding full de-institutionalisation and an enlargement of citizenship for people with mental health problems.

Community Care: Concept and Practice

When the Labour government came to power in 1997, it announced the need for rapid reform of mental health services based on the impression (but no evidence) that 'care in the community has failed' (Dobson, 1998). The term 'community care' has also become something of a catch-all phrase for describing a range of different service

configurations at a variety of historical points. Its original inclusion in
the 1930 Mental Treatment Act was linked essentially to a new move
to voluntary admission (previously all 'lunatics' were certified). After
the Second World War it became a vague euphemism for everything
and anything not provided by the large institutions. However, the con
tinuing focus of what went on in institutions, whether they were being
criticised, defended, emptied or superseded by DGH units, meant that
non-hospital care was hardly considered and planned in a systematic
way. Instead, in practice in the 1970s, 'community care' meant re-
institutionalisation; moving patients to general hospital wards and nursing
homes rather than ordinary community living for people previously
warehoused in the asylums. In particular, medical interests portrayed
DGH units as 'community care', using the argument that the new (and
conveniently more prestigious) hospital base brought care for mental
illness in line with all other types of morbidity in other medical
specialisms. In this context, the 'community' simply meant 'in line
with everybody in the general population'. Thus one version of discourse
about community care was shaped heavily by professional self-interest.

By the 1990s 'community care' had a broad meaning, including the
goal of providing comprehensive outreach, day and residential services and support for ordinary facilities within a locality. In principle
at least 'community care' now extends to social inclusion and the promotion of access to facilities and services used by other people living
in the community and to the rights and responsibilities of participation
in local community activities.

In recent times, then, 'community care' has come to mean several
things. It has been an abstract aspiration upheld by those seeking to
remove oppressive barriers between people with mental health problems and others. It has been a description of service reconfiguration
after the large institutions closed. It has been seen primarily as a cost-
minimisation strategy by the state. It has been depicted by its critics
as a form of neglect and irresponsibility. Moreover, the general term
'community care' describes different things for different client groups:
for example, some groups were institutionalised, and then became de-
institutionalised, on a large scale (people with learning difficulties and
those with mental health problems), but this was not true for people
with physical disabilities or older people, who had always predominantly been at home. Despite this, the recent social administrative
umbrella of 'community care' has tended to cover all of these 'chronic',
'enduring' or 'continuing care' groups.

An early ideological commitment to 'community care' was associated with a vague homely utopianism, prior to it being effected as a practical reality. Titmuss in the 1960s suggested that the notion of community care conjured 'up a sense of warmth and human kindness, essentially personal and comforting' (Titmuss, 1968). This early, positive, view emphasised the idea of leaving the disabling environment of the institution behind and ushering in the enabling possibilities of ordinary living. Such an ideology was elaborated most extensively in relation to learning disabilities under the notion of 'normalisation' (Wolfensberger, 1972) and was subsequently extended to mental health (Ramon, 1991). The essential political problem for government during the 1980s and 1990s about this notion that people with a variety of disabilities had rights of ordinary citizenship was that the central but latent function of the old institution, the social control of risky behaviour, no longer had a site of operation. This is why both Conservative and Labour administrations seriously reviewed the option of legislation and other administrative procedures to minimise risk outside hospital settings. Examples in this regard included the care programme approach and community treatment orders (see later in this chapter and Chapter 12).

Lessons from the End of the Twentieth Century

During the 1980s and 1990s community mental health facilities certainly took practical form, suggesting that Titmuss's points did not remain mere aspirations or rhetoric. However, the adequacy of this practical form remained contentious. On the one hand, its critics wanted less community care and a return to the certainties of hospital segregation. On the other hand, advocates argued that community care had not failed; it had merely not been properly implemented. Thus one answer to concerns about 'the failure of community care' was to re-invest in the old order in relation to the management of madness. The contrary view was that the answer to the problems of community care was not more hospital beds, but more community care.

   In the latter regard, the point made was that residential and day care, community mental health centres and crisis intervention services existed but received poor levels of finance compared with hospitals. The run-down of hospital services and the development of community-based services has presented authorities with the financial and pragmatic difficulties of trying to run both services in tandem. In 1975 the White Paper, *Better Services for the Mentally Ill*, set out norms (which later became guidelines) for future community services. However, mechanisms for monitoring the wide range of community mental health services did not develop adequately. In the absence of the availability of such data, the impression was created that there were few or no community facilities to replace the abolition of hospital beds.

However, systematic attempts to compensate for poor monitoring suggested a more complex picture than either outright success or abject failure for community care. The Audit Commission (1986), taking the norms set out in the 1975 White Paper as the criteria for success, reported that 70 per cent of the hostel or homes targets were met but only 30 per cent of the day centres and 40 per cent of the day hospital targets were achieved. One research study which followed up a cohort of former long-stay patients discharged between 1985 and 1989 showed that they were a residentially non-mobile group. However, in terms of quality of life, unmet needs included inadequate living space, and poor work and leisure opportunities. Less than half of the people followed up were in receipt of formal day-care provision (O'Brien, 1992). A sense of this ambiguous picture about the success or otherwise of community care is indicated below in relation to specific types of community facility.

1 *Residential arrangements.* Whilst the role of the private sector in replacing hospital beds remained a marginal activity, residential facilities were increasingly provided by the private sector. By 1999, 40 per cent of all residential provision for people with long-term mental health problems was in the private sector. Private provision was distributed unevenly with a concentration in southern coastal towns and urban districts. Social services provision remained static or declined. A survey in 1992 suggested that health authorities (alone or in partnership with voluntary organisations) were planning to double their residential provision (Faulkner, 1992).

2 *Specialist community mental health care.* Turning from residence to specialist care, Sayce (1989) found that between 1977 and 1987 community mental health centres leapt in number from 1 to 54. A related expanding phenomenon was the 'community mental health team'. These teams developed unevenly, with some being attached to hospitals and others to community mental health centres. It was recognised that within these types of service the optimal version should include a 24-hours-a-day, seven-days-a-week crisis intervention service. It was also acknowledged by the Royal College of Psychiatrists in 1993, when complaining about pressures on bed occupancy, that outreach work in the community could reduce the

need for hospital admission. This was confirmed by Barnes, Bowl and Fisher (1990), who found that the lowest rates of compulsory admissions to hospital were in those localities providing a comprehensive crisis intervention service. Community-orientated mental health professionals advocated that crisis intervention, residential alternatives to hospital and home-based care should be combined with supported primary care work to minimise the need for hospital admission (Stein and Test, 1980; Falloon and Fadden, 1993).

3   *Social care.* Many community mental health services by the 1990s were jointly funded and managed initiatives between health and social services, although health services provision far outstripped that provided by local authorities. Bridging the gap between these two agencies was difficult. Whilst policy-makers had for many years stressed the need for joint planning (e.g., the Nodder Report of 1980), the successful co-ordination of services often proved elusive in practice. A number of structural and other factors contributed to social service input to, and responsibility for, community mental health work being problematic:

(a)   although local authorities, via their social service departments, were responsible for co-ordinating community care (following the 1990 NHS and Community Care Act), the funding of core mental health services was via the NHS;

(b)   the boundaries of responsibility between social and health care were often unclear, so roles and responsibilities in relation to patients/clients could become a focus of dispute between medical and non-medical workers (the reverse might also apply, with patients being neglected because each party in the social/health split considered that the other was responsible for a service);

(c)   social services were underresourced compared with the NHS.

After 1997 a number of policy directives were issued about reversing this separation between health and social care which we return to in Chapter 12.

The Limitations of Mental Health Care in a Post-Institutional Context

By the mid-1990s the closure of the Victorian mental hospitals was creating a post-institutional context in which the three major *implicit*

functions of a simple segregative solution to madness were becoming
explicit and problematic.

1   What was *care and treatment* to mean outside a hospital context?
2   How was *risky behaviour* to be controlled outside the hospital?
3   How were people with long-term mental health problems now to
     be *housed*?

These three functions are reconsidered in Chapter 11, when we examine how the effectiveness of mental health services is judged. Here we
briefly note their historical significance in the wake of large hospital
closure. Under the old regime, the three functions were carried out on
a single site, which was being rapidly and permanently lost during the
late 1980s and early 1990s.

   Ironically, some of the concerns about the control of risky behaviour in the community which foreshadowed the Care Programme
Approach were highlighted initially by violence in hospitals, rather
than in domestic or public settings. For example, the Spokes Inquiry
followed the killing of a social worker (Isabel Shwartz) in 1984 by a
patient (Sharon Campbell) in Bexley Hospital. It set out the limitations of care discovered and made recommendations about post-discharge
case management (DHSS, 1988). The report noted the lack of any requirement on the part of services to identify vulnerable patients or
provide individualised care plans, and for agencies with responsibilities for mental health to work together. These themes re-emerged
and were elaborated upon during the 1990s.

   For British mental health policy, 1994 was a year of diagnosis about
the three questions noted above. No fewer than ten reports from official policy bodies emerged about the problems of securing efficient
community care for people with mental health problems. In this section
we will summarise points arising from three of these inquiries.

*The report of the inquiry into the care and treatment of Christopher
Clunis (Ritchie, Dick and Lingham, 1994)*

This report was requested by the Chairs of North East and South East
Thames Regional Health Authorities in July 1993 and was submitted
in February 1994. The inquiry examined the way in which services
failed to respond adequately to Christopher Clunis, a young black man
with a diagnosis of paranoid schizophrenia. He stabbed a stranger
(Jonathan Zito) to death on 17 December 1992 at Finsbury Park

underground station in London. Clunis was subsequently committed to Rampton Special Hospital.

The investigation of the service response to Clunis highlighted a number of problems which are relevant to our discussion here of inadequate community support for people with severe mental health problems. A unique aspect of this case was that the widow of the dead man, Jayne Zito, was an experienced psychiatric social worker. Accordingly, despite losing her husband, she retained a strong interest in campaigning for proper community support for patients. The inquiry highlighted a number of features in the case, as set out below:

1 Although Clunis had been in recurrent contact with services since the mid-1980s, there was poor communication by professionals about each admission. In other words, there was a lack of continuity of care (a motif of the case up to the tragic killing). Prior to his becoming violent in the early 1990s neither he nor his family had been given any systematic help or support by either NHS or social service staff.

2 No discharge plans were made for his care in the community under Section 117 of the Mental Health Act. He was often homeless and out of touch with relatives or services. For seven months between September 1988 and April 1989 he was 'lost', with no record being available of his existence anywhere. In June 1989 the first violent incident was recorded, when he attacked the manager of a bed-and-breakfast hostel. This was the first of a series of incidents, mainly involving him threatening or actually carrying out knife attacks on those around him.

3 During the latter part of his psychiatric career, the inquiry discovered further evidence of a fragmented and underresourced system with professionals being ignorant or poorly aware of prior events and the opinions or concerns of others. Between 1987 and 1992 Clunis had been admitted to four major metropolitan psychiatric units, but each of them lost contact with him. A bed in a secure facility was not always readily available when indicated for Clunis during this period. At one point, to save money, he was transferred from a secure to a general psychiatric bed.

4 Despite Clunis making violent attacks with a screwdriver on strangers in public places on two consecutive days in the week before the killing of Jonathan Zito, and the police being given clear evidence about his identity and whereabouts, they failed to make an arrest.

The main lessons from the Clunis case were that:

(a) professional liaison within the NHS, and between it and other agencies such as the police, housing authorities and social services, were inadequate.
(b) Section 117 of the 1983 Mental Health Act was not being implemented, and other strengthening policies, such as the Department of Health's Care Programme Approach (which, incidentally, did not apply in Wales), were not being put into practice properly.
(c) A range of facilities, from secure psychiatric beds to supported housing in the community, were not being resourced properly.
(d) Even when and if services have procedures in place to receive and treat difficult-to-manage people, they failed to deliver long-term support after or between crises.

This inquiry also noted the failure of professionals rationally to appraise dangerousness and the problems of an overreliance on medication, with the consequent neglect or exclusion of personal and social support for patients and their families.

Creating community care (Mental Health Foundation, 1994)

This report was being prepared at the time of the release of the Clunis inquiry Report and concurred with and extended its implications, when submitted in September 1994. The brief of the inquiry commissioned by the Mental Health Foundation (MHF) was to assess the current state of community care for 'people with severe mental illness'. Early on in the MHF Report there was a recognition that the latter term had no official definition. (Mental illness was not defined under the 1983 Mental Health Act.) The inquiry appealed to the Department of Health to provide a working definition. The attempt by the DH to do so produced a rambling and overinclusive response and service commissioners were none the wiser for it. The MHF Report set out a clear value-led position about responding to the needs of people with mental health problems in the community. These were listed as:

• an appropriate place to live
• an adequate income
• a varied social life
• employment and other day activity
• help and support

• respect and trust
• choice and consultation

The report was also clear about separating the needs of patients and those of carers. Also, as well as the citizenship emphasis for patients in the list above, the report noted that 'Everyone should be able to have a sense of safety in the community.'

The problem checklist it offered pointed the finger firmly at central government and even stipulated that the Prime Minister should take the lead regarding a comprehensive strategy, the provision of sufficient resources and organisational change. The report also noted two other major problems: a lack of understanding of mental illness and diffuse responsibility across agencies. The latter observation could be read as both a traditional lament about professionals not communicating well with each other (as exemplified by the Clunis case) and as a governmental failure to engender co-operation and collaboration. Governments during the 1990s, when faced with criticisms of community care policies, tended to stress the failure of professionals to collaborate and liaise properly. However, both the Clunis and MHF inquiries complained of the failure of central government to give a clear lead to local services about strategy. At times there had been confusing guidance issued about the implementation of three overlapping policies, which separately and together were not working efficiently: Section 117 of the 1983 Mental Health Act; the Care Programme Approach; and care management. The confusion these created at a local level was compounded by the introduction of supervision registers. The MHF inquiry recommended that people placed on supervision registers should have access to an advocate. Four years after this, when the Scoping Exercise about new mental health legislation took place, a similar point about advocacy being a balance against coercion was made (see Chapter 12).

In the wake of the 1990 Community Care and NHS Act, and until Labour reformed the internal market after 1998, the issues of lack of organisational stability and inadequate resources together were traceable to central government policies: marketisation, and shifting responsibility for community care to local authorities, without providing them with the financial support to operate a needs-led service. These led to an uneasy, patchy and faltering transition to a community-based system of care. Inadequate co-ordinated joint commissioning of care between local and health authorities was one problem the MHF inquiry highlighted.

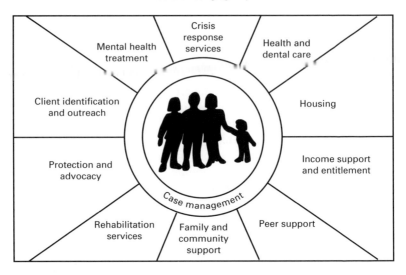

FIGURE 9.1 *The elements of an appropriate community service*

Source: Strathdee, personal communication (1995).

Overall, the MHF Report combined a critique of the then government's lack of mental health policy strategy with an attempt to offer positive advice to purchasers and providers about making the best of resources. Its view of an integrated mental health service can be seen in Figure 9.1.

The holistic picture offered in Figure 9.1 still has relevance today as a template for judging the adequacy of community mental health care development in any locality.

Finding a Place *(Audit Commission, 1994)*

This constituted a critical overview of the success of government mental health policy. It is not clear from the report whether this was an intended or an unintended consequence. Either way, Conservative health ministers indicated their profound irritation with its analysis, probably for the following reasons. First, the report (like that from the MHF) held the government responsible for a lack of clear vision of, and responsibility for, a co-ordinated mental health strategy. Second, it told the government how it could save money to advance community developments: by implication, a cost-sensitive administration was not doing its job properly. Third, it referred to the backlash against community care created by events such as the fatal stabbing of Jonathan Zito. Former Health Secretary Virginia Bottomley was pointedly cited (but not supported) as complaining that 'the pendulum has swung too far' (Audit Commission, 1994, 7). Fourth, given these three features of the report, its overall message was very negative about government success.

By contrast, health ministers had been keen to emphasise how much thought, care and resources they had put into community care. Examples of this that were regularly cited by Virginia Bottomley and her junior minister John Bowis were statements on the increase in the number of specialist staff (especially CMHNs) and those emphasising supervision registers. *Finding a Place* pointedly queries whether the skill mix of community nursing staff was appropriate and cost-efficient. Also, claims by the government that they held the strategic reins about mental health were disingenuous. The overall welfare policy since 1979 has been about devolving blame to local authorities, whilst withholding the resources required for them to take responsibility for efficient community services. The role of central government had been to lay down the law occasionally, metaphorically in relation to registers and literally in relation to the stronger community supervision orders. But such sporadic shows of authoritarianism did not constitute strategic leadership.

Finding a Place was a detailed appraisal of current services. Even a summary is beyond the scope of our space here, but some of its key points or features are set out below:

1 Two-thirds of the £1.8 billion spent on mental health in 1992/3 went to inpatient facilities.
2 Given that community mental health services are more cost-effective and preferred by users and their relatives, a strategy needed to be put in place to break the inertia about inpatient work.
3 Government should be more directive about rebalancing resources. Some districts needed more money than others (especially the large urban areas containing inner-city problems). These needed some resource allocations taken from other localities.
4 Savings could be made to move forward on community developments in a number of ways:

   (a) by employing unqualified staff to carry out tasks currently being done by more expensive trained staff in the community;

(b) by the reduction in bed use being accompanied by more efficient home-based assessments and treatment, which would lead
to fewer admissions and shorter stays in hospital;
(c) by reducing the current overutilisation of 24-hour-staffed accommodation.

Sub-point (a) above relates to the finding of the inquiry that expensive
and highly trained CMHNs were carrying out work that could have
been done by less qualified people. In some cases CPNs were also
found to be failing to prioritise those with the most severe needs.

The savings suggested in the report by these three measures (per
annum, at the time of costing in 1992/3) would have been: £100 million from a 12 per cent reduction in inpatient services; £42.5 million
from rationalising accommodation staffing; and £13.3 million from
changing the community nursing skill mix. Thus, over £155 million
could have been reinvested in improving community care by this formula. By avoiding demands for *extra* resources (the emphasis of the
MHF report), *Finding a Place* paradoxically posed a threat to government authority. Conservative administrations, since 1979, had been used
to warding off (often with pride) opposition demands for more public
spending.

A series of points raised by the MHF report were also made by the
Audit Commission. These included the need for collaboration with
housing authorities; caution about resources leaking from hospital closures away from mental health facilities; making care programming
work efficiently; and the responsibilities of local purchasers and providers to improve collaboration and liaison about assessing and responding
to needs. The shared responsibility of local authorities, health purchasers,
NHS trusts, GP fund-holders and statutory providers was highlighted.
The report endorsed the concept of a comprehensive set of activities
to respond to the range of needs of people with mental health problems.

Together, these three reports highlighted and analysed some of the
difficulties that community care was encountering in the mid-1990s.
The fate of these debates in the late 1990s is picked up in Chapter 12.

Community Care, Medication and Risk Management

The shift to community settings has exposed a new set of debates about
the limitations of, and cautions about, major tranquillisers as a form of
treatment. Anti-psychotic medication has been viewed as the main means

of containing the symptoms of mental health problems in the community. Thus one common concern of clinicians and policy-makers alike has been to ensure compliance by people with a diagnosis of psychosis with their prescribed medication. However, the 'older' anti-psychotics (the 'major tranquillisers' or 'neuroleptics') which are still in common use have side-effects which also impact on recipients' quality of life. When major tranquillisers were first introduced in the late 1950s they were given in low doses. Subsequently, dose levels increased until, by the 1970s, the limitations of these drugs became apparent. In particular, iatrogenic tardive dyskinesia – the drug-induced movement disorders – emerged as a hazard for psychiatric patients. Instead of being used in low doses and on a temporary basis, it became commonplace for major tranquillisers to be used at high doses and permanently, using maintenance depot injections. The risk of tardive dyskinesia increases with both dose level and chronicity of use.

The disabling impacts of these drugs were, until recently, contained in hospital settings. Now they are experienced in the community. Patients themselves may be hampered by the iatrogenic effects of drugs, and their stigma in the eyes of others will be made greater by the effects. Major tranquillisers have a dual disabling effect. They impair concentration and volition and so pose problems for people in daily living. Also, the disfiguring movement disorders they trigger make their recipients very obvious to those around them. This increases perceptions of difference or oddity in the eyes of non-patients. The stigma of having a psychiatric diagnosis is then amplified by the iatrogenic physical impact of psychiatric treatment. The new anti-psychotics have less disabling effects; however, these drugs are not universally used and matters of cost-effectiveness have retarded their widespread availability to patients on the NHS.

Tardive dyskinesia in patients living in the community is only one part of the iatrogenic problem. The adverse effects of neuroleptics pose a dilemma for those responsible for the development and implementation of mental health policy. This is particularly so in a cultural context which is becoming increasingly sensitive to risk (Giddens, 1991). On the one hand, people with a diagnosis of schizophrenia are often portrayed in the media and in the public imagination as potentially violent. The official reports discussed above emphasise strategies which ensure that patients receive medication as the means of preventing violent acts. On the other hand, emerging concerns about the iatrogenic effects of neuroleptics (Brown and Funk, 1986), together with the evolution of consumer-orientated approaches to health care which promise to give due regard to patients' views of services and treatment, make the risks associated with neuroleptic therapy less acceptable. Somehow, policy-makers have to steer a path which reflects sensitivities about both these sources of risk.

With the closure of large mental health hospitals, more psychotic patients have become visible in public spaces. Although psychiatry extended its remit from madness to include neurosis after the First World War, the continued use of Victorian asylums during most of this century separated one psychiatric sub-population ('psychotics') from another living in the community ('neurotics'). The physical separation of these groups has been replaced increasingly with a conceptual separation. The recent shifts in mental health policy have been associated with a different public and mass media response to these two groups. The recipients of minor tranquillisers became the focus of consumer campaigning and attracted substantial public and media sympathy (Bury and Gabe, 1990). By contrast, the media attention on madness has been about dangerousness and threat. Those diagnosed as being schizophrenic are just as (if not more) prone to iatrogenic risk when receiving major rather than minor tranquillisers, but they receive little public sympathy. Thus the social problem associated with neurotic distress has been psychiatric *treatment*, whereas the social problem associated with madness has been psychiatric *patients*.

The Theory and Practice of British Case Management and the Care Programme Approach

Prior to the 'year of diagnosis' we mentioned above (1994), the British government had introduced an overarching framework aimed at the systematic co-ordination of case management for those entering specialist mental health services. The care programme approach (CPA) was introduced in 1991. It contained four key elements:

- arrangements for assessing the health and social needs of recipients of specialist mental health services
- the regular use of a care plan that identified which provider was responsible for different aspects of a person's care
- a key worker who would monitor and co-ordinate care for the individual
- regular review and (as appropriate) changes to the care plan.

Since the introduction of CPA, 'tiered' prioritisation of patients and the identification of patients at risk through supervision registers have also been required (DH, 1995). The idea was that all patients in contact with services would be subject to CPA but that some would require greater scrutiny and service input. The Labour government inherited this formula in 1997 and continued to endorse it as the mainstay of good quality community-based management for psychotic patients, despite the concept of community care being problematised by health ministers, and controversial cases such as that of Christopher Clunis. In 1997 approximately 1 per cent of the total population of England was subject to CPA, of whom about 1 per cent was included in local supervision registers (Bindman *et al.*, 1999).

In 1999 the Department of Health issued a set of suggestions to revise the original CPA concept (DH, 1999b). Not only was *Effective Care Co-ordination in Mental Health Services* sub-titled *Modernising the Care Programme Approach*, but the text acknowledged problems with the use of CPA to date. It was noted that CPA was experienced as 'over-bureaucratic' by professionals and 'confusing' due to 'lack of consistency' by service managers and users. An important ideological shift in the guidance was the recognition that case management should focus not on diagnosis but on need, vulnerability and risk. Confirmation of problems with the implementation of CPA was further suggested by a national evaluation of CPA based on measures of population mental health need. The evaluation found that prioritisation to receive specialist mental health services was carried out inconsistently when applied to criteria of need and risk (which were also poorly defined). This suggested that there was also an inequitable use of resources (Bindman *et al.*, 1999).

A major problem that CPA faced was that the concept (the four elements noted above) was eminently sensible as a broad strategy but was without reference to the vagaries of actual practice. For example, when professionals experienced the system as 'over-bureaucratic' they would be half-hearted about its implementation. In many localities it deteriorated into a box-ticking exercise and was not delivered according to its original spirit. The most damning problem though for CPA was that it did not specify what good community mental health care was, as a set of clinical not administrative practices. What if, even when CPA was properly implemented, there was merely the aggregate of ineffective or dubious service inputs? This empirical question was soon to be relevant as research on intensive case management in Britain did not clearly support the position that CPA led to raised levels of service efficiency as judged by fewer hospital admissions (Bindman *et al.*, 1999; Burns *et al.*, 1999; Marshall, Bond and Stein, 1999). Indeed when the typical inputs to mental health services are contrasted with the successful intense case management (Assertive Community Treatment, or ACT) evaluated in the USA, then levels of both intensity and complexity of service inputs are demonstrably inferior in Britain (Allness and Knoedler, 1999).

In the USA co-ordinated assertive outreach does not merely signal low case loads (as in Britain) but the systematic co-ordination of multiple treatment inputs. In the US model their notion of intense case management in the community is 14 service contacts per week utilising up to 12 different staff. British community mental health workers do not typically reach this level of activity. The US model also seeks to combine medication, social skills training, family psycho-educational methods, supportive counselling, cognitive behaviour therapy, group therapy and supported employment. Thus the staffing levels and the service processes are not typically matched in Britain. Whereas comparisons of standard with intense care in British CMHTs reveals little difference in client outcomes, reviews of fully implemented ACT in the USA and Australia show significant superiority for the ACT model. Thus the problem with the British reliance on CPA has been that it has emphasised an *administrative* system for community mental health work but it has not defined in any detail at all a form of optimal *clinical practice.*

Community Care and 'Mild to Moderate' Mental Health Problems

A final point to note about the shifting discourse about community-based psychiatric populations is the expanding remit of professionals for 'minor' psychiatric illnesses which we noted in Chapter 8. With the increased detection of anxiety and depression in primary care settings, and a commitment of the Royal Colleges of Psychiatrists and General Practitioners to 'beat depression', the psychiatrisation of the community has become substantial. Community psychiatric epidemiology is now identifying large groups in the population, particularly women, as suffering from some form of psychiatric morbidity. From this perspective, 'worry', 'anxiety' and 'stress' are symptoms affecting, it seems, a large minority of the British population. It is not clear at the time of writing how far this psychiatrisation of hitherto everyday distress will be taken. Policy questions are raised by this enthusiasm for detection, which may, in part, be seen as an attempt to find a new role for professionals such as psychiatrists whose traditional roles are changing and being challenged by other stakeholders. If such large numbers in the general population are deemed to be psychologically distressed, what is to be done? How will attaching a psychiatric label to distress, which cannot easily be separated from social circumstances (Pilgrim and Bentall, 1998), help those people and affect the other informal means by which people resolve or cope with problems in everyday life? Will they all be given medication or offered counselling? If not, how will decisions be made to prioritise need within a health service so conscious now of cost containment? If rationing is to take place, what criteria will be used and who will be charged with responsibility for their implementation? As we note later in Chapter 12, mental health policy may still be centred on 'severe mental illness' or 'severe and enduring mental health problems'; however, mental health promotion and the treatment of anxiety and depression solely in primary care have also become part of the official agenda of government.

Conclusion

This chapter has explored the recent discourse about community mental health work. It is clear that this has innumerable implicit as well as explicit meanings, so that 'community care' can no longer be a simple shorthand term which a variety of disparate parties can use with a common sense of confidence. Notwithstanding Frank Dobson's unwise statement, community care has not definitely failed as a policy. However, it not been operating for a long enough period of time to judge whether it can be defined as a success in a way which would satisfy all parties interested in mental health. The best we can say at present is that mental health care in a post-institutional world has opened up a new set of debates about the amelioration of distress and dysfunction, the control or tolerance of madness, and the promotion of well-being. It also raises a set of questions about citizenship for those who are disabled on a temporary or enduring basis by their mental health problems and the degree to which state-funded services can intervene positively in this regard. These and other questions will be discussed in the next two chapters.

10

The Disappearing Institution?

Introduction

This chapter returns to the enduring legacy of the old asylum system. Whether the focus has been on the purported impact of pharmacological innovations, the fiscal crisis of the state or a shift in psychiatric discourse, most of the arguments of policy analysts suggest a demise of institutional arrangements, and their predominant displacement by community mental health work which we discussed in the preceding chapter. The re-orientation toward community management has been accompanied by changes in the way in which mental health has as a topic been treated by sociology and social policy. Not only has the relevance of inpatient work faded from view in theoretical analyses, compared to past work on the total institution as exemplified by *Asylums* (Goffman, 1961), but a 'post-modern' trend has demoted the political, economic and experiential importance of coercive bio-medical regimes.

However, below we argue that despite developments outside institutions, the role of institutional psychiatry is a strong, albeit changing, feature of mental health policy and practice. The historical, organisational or policy focus of contributors such as Erving Goffman, Andrew Scull and Philip Bean still have importance in understanding the configuration of contemporary mental health services and management. We first look at the shift in theoretical accounts which have accompanied the demise of the large institutions. We then go on to examine the way in which mental health practice still, to a large degree, revolves around institutions and admissions. We argue that this evidence still needs to be accommodated within an analysis of the institutions, albeit modified, from earlier sociological and policy accounts.

The rise of post-modern accounts of mental health practice and policy

Accounts about the rise and grip of the British asylum system in the nineteenth century, humanistic analyses of the everyday life of psychiatric patients as an oppressed group, and exploration of professional interests and those of significant others in conspiratorial collusion (Goffman's 'betrayal funnel'), formed an influential backdrop to deinstitutionalisation. With the physical demise of the total institution there has also been the collapse of totalising theory in the shift towards post-modernism in sociology which has produced more fragmented accounts about particular topics and a strong shift of interest to *productive power*. This emphasis in Foucault's later work about the 'psy complex' and conversational treatments, which are 'anxiously sought and gratefully received', now places the focus on selfhood being inscribed upon its subjects by mental health work (Ingleby, 1983; Rose, 1990; Parker *et al.*, 1995). The post-modern focus on the production or inscription of subjective life by the technologies of the self – especially the discursive practices of counselling and psychotherapy – contrasts with older anti-psychiatric concerns about coercion and repression. This is put succinctly by Miller and Rose (1988, 174): 'We argue that it is more fruitful to consider the ways that regulatory systems have sought to promote subjectivity than to document ways in which they have crushed it.'

Despite the stimulating utility of this type of analysis, institutional psychiatry and its repressive role in society still requires consideration. Common sense might lead us to conclude that, with the closure of large mental hospitals, such arrangements are indeed simply a thing of the past. However, there are strong indications that this *socio*logical and *logical* concurrence is undermined by a number of considerations which will be summarised under the following headings: safety and dangerousness; evidence of increased compulsory admission; professional inertia; and users' accounts of services and community living.

Safety and dangerousness

By 'institutional psychiatry', we mean a constellation of organisational features: hospital-based activities and routines; lawful state-delegated repressive power; bio-medical problem formulation and intervention; and an implicit or explicit organisational emphasis upon the control of risky behaviour. Mental health policy, *since* active hospital run-down was formalised and effected, reflects enduring governmental concern about the social control of madness. The latter was the focus of humanistic anti-institutional critiques pre-dating de-institutionalisation. The last British Conservative government introduced supervision registers and supervised discharge between 1994 and 1996. Despite its broad rhetoric about social inclusion, when the Labour government arrived in 1997 it did not emphasise a policy of enlarged citizenship for psychiatric patients. It focused instead on public safety and the need to introduce legislation forcibly to remove people from their homes who were refusing to comply voluntarily with medication regimes to a clinical setting. As we noted in the previous chapter, Frank Dobson, the Secretary of state for Health, argued that:

> Care in the community has failed. Discharging people from institutions has brought benefits to some. But it has left many vulnerable patients trying to cope on their own. Others have been left to become a danger to themselves and a nuisance to others. Too many confused and sick people have been left wandering the streets and sleeping rough. A small but significant minority have become a danger to the public as well as themselves. (Dobson, 1998)

The full new policy, which this statement launched (DH, 1998), was entitled *Modernising Mental Health Services: Safe, Sound and Supportive* (see Chapter 12). It reflected in its sub-title the priorities of government, with safety being first and support being last. This leads to a highly contradictory document which, on the one hand, advocates the reversal of stigma and discrimination but, on the other, emphasises public safety. Moreover, the investment announced related mainly to more acute inpatient facilities, especially more medium secure beds. This reinforced a trend in services during the 1990s of more and more locked wards being established, usually under the euphemistic cover of 'intensive care' or 'special care'. Proposed changes to the Mental Health Act (to be discussed further in Chapter 12), announced at the end of 1999, called for an extension of powers to coercive treatment in the community. If this is effected, it will allow easier return to hospital with less formality. Adoption of more restrictive civil commitment criteria and procedures internationally as well as nationally have undermined the countervailing policy trajectory of voluntary therapeutic relationships. At times this has led to new alliances in which clinicians have joined voices with patient groups opposed to coercive treatment (Bracken and Thomas, 1998; Hiday *et al.*, 1999).

Thus in many ways recent mental health policy does *not* reflect the post-modern agenda about voluntary relationships, 'minor' mental health problems and the production rather than the repression of selfhood. Instead, it continues to place centre-stage responses to the threat which embodied irrationality (unintelligible conduct) poses to a social, economic and moral order. In this respect, it could be argued that little has changed in a hundred years. What seems to have happened is that the three main functions of the old total institution (care, control and accommodation) are now being reconstructed by a set of interweaving social policies. These combine acute DGH psychiatric units, community services (assertive outreach and community mental health teams), resettlement arrangements and new legislation to enable surveillance and control to take place outside hospitals. The last item on this list is reflected in the policy initiatives mentioned earlier that have occurred since 1994 and have been backed up by government directives and legislation. Examples of this are supervision registers, supervised discharge, the CPA and, recently, the review of the 1983 Mental Health Act to adapt to service arrangements in the wake of large hospital closures.

Evidence of increased compulsory admission

An important consequence of large hospital closures has been that the continuing coercive institutional role of psychiatry has been associated with a crisis in the physical capacity of the DGH inpatient unit. The latter has increasingly become a crucible for frenetic social control. In a study of a range of inpatient units (Sainsbury Centre, 1998), the following points were emphasised when summarising official data from a range of sources on British inpatient work.

1   The number of psychiatric beds declined from 155 000 in the mid-1950s to 37 000 in the mid-1990s, with 22 000 being in DGH units.
2   Between 1986 and 1996 the throughput of beds doubled to 5.7 patients per bed per year.
3   Between 1983 and 1994 admissions increased from 200 000 to 270 000 per year.
4   Officially recorded levels of coercively detained patients increased from 8 per cent in the early 1980s to 32 per cent in the late 1990s (with a range of 4 per cent to 37 per cent across localities).
5   Bed pressures have increased on open wards because of the increase in admission of those warranting medium secure provision,

an increased incidence of drug and alcohol related problems and court diversion schemes to keep people with a diagnosis of mental illness out of prison. Also, even though about a quarter of in-patients were deemed not to require hospital residence in 1997, a third lacked access to adequate housing and a quarter lacked access to adequate community support thus delayed discharge compounds the pressure.

6 89 per cent of admissions are on an emergency basis, with one in ten patients being admitted for 'social reasons' (see discussion point below).

7 By 1997 bed occupancy rates of units varied from 86 per cent to 140 per cent. Higher levels of occupancy are found mainly (but not exclusively) in inner-city areas.

In 1997 this picture of intense DGH activity was confirmed by a one-day census carried out by the Mental Health Act Commission and the Sainsbury Centre for Mental Health. This found that most acute wards reported 99 patient residents for every 100 beds available, with 36 per cent of wards reporting more patients than beds. The latter, apparently untenable, feature is explained by patients being present in eccentric arrangements (e.g., mattresses on floors or the use of seclusion rooms as temporary bedrooms).

Point 6 above raises questions of interpretation of what constitutes 'social reasons'. This administrative description is common within mental health work. It tends to refer to people who are homeless or difficult to place, rather than those who are 'just mentally ill'. However, Bean (1980) argues persuasively that *all* psychiatric crises are social crises. That is, 'acute mental illness' which warrants hospitalisation (according to doctors and social workers) reflects a breakdown in the capacity of a familial or other open social system to cope with and contain deviance. As Coulter (1973) demonstrated, professional judgements about the need to admit tend to rubber stamp lay decisions already made about madness by exasperated relatives who seek professional interventions.

Admission pressures on DGH units are coming from displaced volume from the prison service and forensic psychiatric sector (especially medium secure units). On the other side, an underdeveloped community infrastructure means that, despite increased throughput, many patients are being detained in an overly restrictive environment because of insufficient volume in housing stock range and aftercare arrangements. This crisis has led for demands for more resources for inpatient units, which the government is now partially responding to in its new policy noted above. Although the rhetorical emphasis upon community care may have overshadowed inpatient care in government policies in the last 20 years, in *economic terms* the state still emphasises inpatient beds. By 1994, for example, two-thirds of the budget for mental health in England and Wales was spent on acute inpatient facilities (Audit Commission, 1994). A similar health economic conclusion was drawn in 1997, when the average cost to the state of a weekly inpatient stay was calculated to be £924 per resident (Netten and Dennet, 1997).

The picture above from the Sainsbury Centre's reports about activity in acute facilities during the late 1990s was reinforced when the Department of Health released monitored data about admissions under the 1983 Mental Health Act between 1988 and 1999, which are summarised below (DH, 1999a).

1   Formal admissions to hospitals under the 1983 Mental Health Act rose more than 60 per cent from 16 000 in the year 1988–89 to 27 100 in 1998–99.
2   There was a threefold increase in Section 3 admissions (for treatment lasting up to 6 months) from 2800 in 1988–89 to 9200 in 1998–99. This rate reflects a 47 per cent increse in admissions for women and nearly a doubling of the male rate of detention.
3   In the year 1998–99 a total of 20 500 who were admitted originally as informal patients were subsequently compulsorily detained during their hospital stay.

Inpatient services also have to manage a new set of problems which reinforces the role of the institution rather than diminishes it. During periods of community living, revolving door patients are more prone to take recreational drugs, opiates and alcohol than when chronic patients were segregated semi-permanently in the asylum system, with its strict abstinent, quasi-monastic ethos. One consequence has been that psychiatry has medicalised the outcome of the new problem of overlapping deviance as 'dual diagnosis'. With the growth in illicit drug use and the steady increase in alcohol consumption in groups chronically excluded from the labour market, psychiatric patients are now characterised more and more by these addictive problems. Moreover, with bed levels in acute units being much reduced compared to the old asylums, this alters admission criteria in favour of prioritising the control of risky behaviour (harm to self or others). Whilst discharged patients who abstain from alcohol and opiates are actually less dangerous than their non-psychiatric neighbours in community settings, the 'dual diagnosis' group manifests a significantly higher level of violence (Link and Stueve, 1998). Moreover, suicide and parasuicide levels in and out of hospital are high amongst people with enduring mental health problems. This shift of emphasis upon risk has led to more and more patients being detained forcibly, and so the old coercive tradition of institutional psychiatry continues to be reinforced.

Professional inertia

During the twentieth century it is certainly true that psychiatry became more eclectic in its treatment approaches compared to its Victorian roots. The shellshock problem of the First World War, morale problems and selection in the Second and the post-war legacy of the therapeutic community movement and social psychiatry all engendered, or were associated with, a shift from a narrow and rigid bio-determinism. Psychiatry incorporated first psychoanalytical and then social models. However, this twentieth-century psychiatric eclecticism continued (and continues) to remain heavily biologically-biased. During the 1960s and 1970s 'anti-psychiatry' was still provoked into being, or made possible, by institutional psychiatry.

By the 1990s psychiatric patients were still reporting that the treatment they received was overwhelmingly biological (medication and ECT: Rogers, Pilgrim and Lacey, 1993). In the last ten years in the British NHS there has even been a resurgence of psychosurgery and ECT. During the 1990s, the drug companies have successfully marketed more and more psychotropic products, such as new anti-depressants and anti-psychotic agents. Research grants from bodies such as the Medical Research Council have prioritised biological research, including new forms of CNS photography and post-mortem brain slicing. All this has occurred in spite of the rise of the users' movement, with its opposition to biological psychiatry and its demand for more talking treatments. The persistence of a biological emphasis in psychiatry is not inevitably linked to inpatient regimes and coercive interventions (e.g., anti-depressants are commonplace in primary care, as were the benzodiazepine minor tranquillisers before them). However, the emphasis is compatible with the traditions of ward-based routines, even if those wards are now in small DGH units rather than in the large Victorian asylum. Drugs can be given readily against the will of the patient and so can be used to sedate disruptive individuals and thus quell their social threat. This type of use of 'PRN' ('when required') psychotropic medication is common on acute psychiatric wards, especially directly in the wake of admission.

Whilst it is true that talking treatments embedded in therapeutic community regimes are also compatible with repressive residential settings such as prisons, they are virtually absent from acute psychiatry because they require a stable and selected population. The rapid turnover in DGH units does not provide these conditions and so medication routines continue to dominate their functioning. Medication can be offered or imposed impersonally and immediately to strangers and short-term or long-term stayers alike. By contrast, psychological approaches require a period of sustained social contract and mutual personal commitment between patients and their therapists.

The professional socialisation of the two core professions of psychiatry and mental health nursing is still predominantly in hospital settings. Most trained psychiatrists are then employed in hospitals, with a few working full time in Community Mental Health Teams. More nurses work in inpatient settings than in the community. Even in more community-orientated professions, such as occupational therapy and clinical psychology, mental health placements during training are often in acute psychiatric units.

As far as psychiatry's continuing repressive role is concerned, it is significant that debates about coercive powers in community settings have brought a mixed response from the profession. For ethical and practical reasons the profession was split about mooted Community Treatment Orders in the late 1980s. The same is true of current debates about new community powers with the incipient replacement of the 1983 Mental Health Act. A minority of radical psychiatrists are using the opportunity to argue for the uncoupling of their treatment role from their social control role (Bracken and Thomas, 1999). On the other side there continue to be psychiatrists who have been in favour of minimising legal limits on what they see as their ability to treat people and who consequently express few qualms about their coercive role in or out of inpatient settings. This paternalistic emphasis on the 'right to treat' is a continuation of an ethos which displaced an earlier moral concern about the citizen's fundamental right to liberty (Bean, 1980). That is, a substantial number of mental health professionals continue to formulate their coercive role by arguing that they are offering 'treatment under the Mental Health Act' in a way which outweighs or obscures the right to liberty of those receiving their diagnoses.

The possibility of a more eclectic 'biopsychosocial' approach (Clare,

1976; Goldberg and Huxley, 1980; Falloon and Fadden, 1988) is more evident in community mental health work than in an inpatient culture because the coercive element in the interface with patients is largely absent. This frees up community-based workers to emphasise voluntary supportive interventions with clients, in which their psycho-social needs are identified and attended to. The emergence of Community Mental Health Centres and Community Mental Health Teams during the 1980s has created a new sub-system of mental health work which is isolated from the inpatient culture. Community mental health nurses and community support workers working outside the hospital setting tend, like their inpatient colleagues, to develop their own separate preferred ways of working. Even in community work, though, a bio-medical inertia is evident. For example, community mental health nurses still typically carry through medically-prescribed treatments, such as depot injections of major tranquillisers for those with a diagnosis of schizophrenia.

Users' accounts of services and community living

The accounts which psychiatric patients give of their life in the community and their service contact provides evidence of a different sort of influence of hospital-based practices on their lives. There is evidence to suggest that their lives outside hospital are dominated by the centralising focus of hospital-based mental health practice (Pilgrim and Hoser, 1999). A key point in this report was that although the patients surveyed spent most of their time outside hospital, their main preoccupations were with their local DGH acute psychiatric units. Similarly, the relatives (who were surveyed separately) also focused their attention on complaints about DGH care. The difference between the two groups was that the relatives wanted the inpatient regime to be both more controlling and more therapeutic. The patients only wanted the latter. Compared to wider concerns about improved citizenship in the community, the respondents were preoccupied with inpatient care. This was described as unimaginative, lacking in treatment options beyond medication and ECT and with low staff–patient interaction.

Conclusion

These reflections on the inertia of institutional psychiatry point to a fundamental feature of contemporary mental health work. The old hospitals may have now virtually disappeared, but inpatient regimes with coercive bio-medical routines still predominate in terms of routine clinical practices and government investment in beds. Moreover, acute DGH units are not the only manifestation of this point. The Special Hospital system still exists, as does a network of regional medium secure units. As was noted earlier, the Labour government elected in 1997 intends to expand the latter. Moreover, even if psychiatric bed levels have dropped dramatically in the last 20 years, inpatient regimes still dominate the consciousness of those outside hospital. Thus the hospital remains centre-stage as a physical space and discursive influence in mental health policy.

11

Questions of Effectiveness

Introduction

In Chapter 3 we noted that, during Victorian period, mad-doctors and lay administrators of asylums generated a rhetoric of therapeutic optimism in which they made inflated claims of cure. Since then, a dilemma which has dogged those professionally responsible for madness and psychological distress relates to their credibility. Put simply, what can be reasonably expected of mental health professionals? This is a global question for governments, since they all need to contain expenditure on health and social services. Cost minimisation or cost-effectiveness have become hallmarks of health service management throughout the world.

This chapter examines the effectiveness of mental health services and the problems created by them pursuing aims which are at times contradictory. Because this latter point is central to the question of effectiveness, we address it first below.

Effective at what?

The aims of the mental health industry require careful consideration. Are services in the business primarily of *curing* or symptomatically ameliorating mental illness? This question is only meaningful to those who consider that mental illness is a coherent concept which can be operationalised into therapeutic targets, and not all parties agree on this supposition. Alternatively, is mental health work about *controlling* the disruptive, burdensome, anxiety-inducing or threatening behavioural outcome of psychological abnormality? Given the extensive considerations given in legislation (see Chapters 3 and 12) to the conditions under which madness can be lawfully contained and regulated by agents of the State, the mental health industry has always been in large part a site of coercive social control. This role is not always conceded explicitly. For example, some professionals believe that they are merely treating illness in those who, through lack of insight, require paternalistic care. Psychiatrists may find it easier to think of 'treating people under the Mental Health Act' than accept that they are agents of social control employed by the State to regulate one particular aspect of deviance.

Another consideration is this: do mental health services enhance or diminish the quality of life of patients? This question has arisen more recently because of the rise in consumerism in Western democracies. Users of health and welfare services are now encouraged to identify those aspects of service contact or intervention which they found useful and life-enhancing. Related questions about quality of life include the following. Do mental health services improve or jeopardise aspects of citizenship such as employment rights and improved accommodation? Do their social relationships enlarge or diminish in the wake of service contact? These questions about quality of life are important. Indeed some social psychiatrists argue that the ultimate measure of service efficiency should be the outcome of improved quality of life (Brugha and Lindsey, 1996).

We can see that the question of effectiveness can only be answered if we operationalise what the *aims* of the mental health industry are. In this chapter the three main criteria we set out above will be examined in the following order.

1 Do services *cure* or effectively ameliorate the symptoms of mental illness?
2 Do services effectively *improve the quality of life* of patients?
3 Do services effectively *control risky behaviour?*

We would argue that mental health services currently can be judged by answering these three questions. We would also emphasise that success in one domain may lead to failure in another (Pilgrim, 1997). For example, a service which is highly efficient at controlling risky behaviour may, as a result, pay less attention to ameliorating symptoms and may impact negatively on a patient's quality of life. This and other contradictions may be one reason why mental health services are so controversial at times and why staff feel that they are often playing a 'no win' game. At the end of this chapter we will return to these contradictions.

In 1998 the British government announced its plan to improve the efficiency of the NHS (see chapter 12. The policy (of 'clinical governance') had five main building blocks: quality; clinical effectiveness; risk assessment and management; audit; and continuous professional development. This chapter will touch on all of these and focus in particular on the first three. In order to highlight the problematic nature of treatment, risk management and quality of life enhancement, we will introduce a summary of the criticisms of the ways in which women and black people experience mental health services.

Do Services Cure or Effectively Ameliorate the Symptoms of Mental Illness?

This question can be broken down into four others.

1　Is the question meaningful to all parties?
2　What evidence exists about treatment effectiveness?
3　What evidence exists that services engender cost-effective treatment?
4　What evidence exists that treatments are offered equitably?

These four questions will now be addressed in turn.

Is the question meaningful to all parties?

This begged question may seem to be pernickety or pedantic but it has a daily and political relevance. The general legislative framework present in most countries operates on the assumption that 'mental illness' (and 'mental disorder', which in addition subsumes the more controversial category of 'personality disorder') has a non-problematic factual status. However, this legislative consensus does not have the agreement of all stakeholders. Many users of services do not see themselves as being mentally ill. Rogers, Pilgrim and Lacey (1993) found that only 10 per cent of psychiatric patients surveyed viewed their difficulties as being as a result of mental illness. The mental health service users' movement is divided over the status of mental illness, with some accepting psychiatric diagnoses in principle and others rejecting their legitimacy (Pilgrim and Rogers, 1991).

　　Professionals too are divided. Szasz (1962), a psychiatrist and psychoanalyst, offered a seminal critique of the concept of mental illness, arguing that minds, like economies but unlike bodies, could only be sick metaphorically, not literally. Other professionals elaborated versions of the Szaszian position about the 'myth of mental illness'. Clinical psychologists are ambivalent about the status of mental illness. Whilst some investigate the 'psychological treatment of schizophrenia', others argue that specific categories such as 'schizophrenia' or 'depression' are, for scientific purposes, all but useless (Bentall, Jackson and Pilgrim, 1988; Pilgrim and Bentall, 1999). Politicians have been so unconcerned about the conceptual status of mental illness that they have rarely bothered to define it in legislation. Under the 1983 Act it is left undefined. It thus comes to mean in practice whatever professionals say it is. In policy debates politicians and their civil servants tend to evade problems of conceptual contestation, leaving them unresolved and ambiguous.

What is the evidence for treatment effectiveness?

One common agreement is that even if mental illness, and the diagnoses it subsumes, are medical reifications, specific 'symptoms' or 'presenting problems' are not. Even Szasz and other critics of psychiatric diagnoses are part of this consensus. All accept that some people hear voices while others do not. All accept that some people fear going out of their house. All accept that some people feel so profoundly miserable that they see little point in continuing to live. In this light, we need to examine what evidence exists about the effectiveness of interventions to reverse these specifiable states.

The literature on this can be divided into that looking at somatic treatments (drugs and ECT) and that looking at conversational treatments (the psychological therapies). In particular these two bodies of literature can be adjudged by two criteria, one related to professional judgements about the symptomatic impact of treatment and the other related to recipient satisfaction. When we appraise the evidence of effectiveness we need to keep both these criteria in mind.

Claims of clinical effectiveness have been made for all of the main current interventions to be found in mental health services: major and minor tranquillisers; ECT; anti-depressants; lithium; and behavioural, cognitive behavioural, psychodynamic and other forms of psychological therapy (Bradley and Hirsch, 1986; Bergin and Garfield, 1994). That is, all these interventions have been demonstrated, using randomised controlled trials, to be effective in reducing psychiatric symptomatology. In relation to the commonest form of treatment for psychotic disorders, neuroleptics, controlled trials have consistently demonstrated that most patients who receive these drugs experience fewer 'positive' symptoms and are hospitalised less often than patients receiving placebos or other kinds of medication (Green, 1988). However, it is only recently that trials have been conducted into the optimum dose levels to control symptoms and prevent relapse. These more recent studies suggest that small dosages of such drugs are as effective, or even more effective, than the higher doses which have generally been prescribed (Bentall *et al.*, 1995). Moreover, some reviewers of the literature on the 'antipsychotics' note that they are highly toxic (Cohen, 1997) and that relapse occurs in two-thirds of medicated patients within a two-year period (Fisher and Greenberg, 1997).

With regard to talking treatments being effective there are particular problems about applying a randomised control trial (RCT) methodology, which has been the main way of assessing the impact of impersonal interventions such as drugs. The RCT model is increasingly being applied to talking treatments (for instance, in the NHS Research and Development initiative on health technologies). It is not that counselling or psychotherapy cannot be assessed in this way; it is that these interventions contain complex personal processes, some of which may be present in ordinary human relationships. If this is the case, then when talking treatments are effective it may be because there is contact with someone who is conversing in a benign, attentive way, rather than it being a reflection of specific technical interventions boosted by a particular therapeutic orientation. This possibility is confirmed by the US research on therapist variables, which demonstrates that there are effective therapists in all therapeutic orientations and that there are wide variations of effectiveness *within* each orientation (Beutler, Machado and Neufeldt, 1994; Dobson and Craig, 1998).

This poses a problem of interpretation about talking treatments. When a drug treatment is compared with a placebo, the *impersonal intervention* can be specified and evaluated. By contrast, psychological technologies (i.e., different approaches to helpful conversations) are mediated necessarily by *personal processes*. This being the case, the latter, rather than the manual-driven detail of the intervention, may account for change. The findings about commonalities across therapies, and similar outcomes achieved, suggest that interpersonal processes may dominate the picture rather than specifiable techniques (Bergin and Garfield, 1994). In this light, whereas a drug treatment can be readily audited in actual services (to check treatment fidelity), with talking treatments it is more difficult to audit the presence of positive features (Pilgrim, 1997).

Despite an overall endorsement of mental health interventions from the RCT clinical literature, a number of recurring problems can be noted, which have been the focus of complaints by recipients of services and contestation from professional researchers. Here we cover six main problems.

(1) Recipients have complained that some treatments have *impaired* their *quality of life*, or have created, as well as solved, problems. Complaints range from the unwanted physiological effects of drugs ('side-effects': see Fisher and Greenberg, 1997) to the sexual and emotional abuse of patients at the hands of psychological therapists (Pilgrim and Guinan, 1999). Moreover, treatments may be experienced as being helpful in some respects but harmful in others (Rogers and Pilgrim, 1994).

(2) Sometimes the degree of iatrogenic damage done by psychiatric treatments has been so profound that their *overall utility* is cast in doubt. For example, benzodiazepines are effective in the short term in reducing anxiety but they are very quickly addictive and ineffective. This has led to recipients needing to seek professional or self-help in withdrawing from their use. Another example is the death rate from major tranquillisers and the widespread prevalence of drug-induced movement disorders (Brown and Funk, 1986). The extent of iatrogenic harm done by psychological therapies has prompted some therapists to argue for the total abolition of their trade (Masson, 1988).

(3) Since psychiatric knowledge is contested by some service-users, and between professionals of differing theoretical orientations, there is *no ready consensus on positive outcome criteria* for interventions. For some people, symptom reduction defines effectiveness. For others (such as a psychodynamic therapist), criteria such as increased insight or even 'therapeutic regression' (getting worse symptomatically) may be deemed to be positive outcomes. Recipients of treatments and other parties may disagree on the utility of interventions. For example, the high non-compliance rates for psychotropic drugs (Kane, 1985) may be contrasted with the enthusiasm that psychiatrists have for their prescription and the concerns that the relatives of patients have for their ensured administration (Finn *et al.*, 1990). Conflicts of opinion and interest about treatment compliance demonstrate that what patients and others consider to be effective is not always the same.

(4) *What is clinically effective may not be cost-effective.* Cost-effective interventions must be clinically effective but not all clinically effective interventions are cost-effective. The earlier examples given about the

merits of selective serotonin re-uptake inhibitor anti-depressants compared to the older tricyclic drugs and the relative costs of psychotherapy
versus counsellor referral in general practice highlight this point.

(5) Overall effectiveness is judged by comparisons between treated
and untreated groups. However, even when treated groups show more
improvement as a whole compared to untreated controls, within the
treated group there will be *some individuals* who *fail to improve* or
who *deteriorate*, and some in the untreated group who improve or fail
to deteriorate. For the former sub-group of treatment 'non-responders',
iatrogenic costs of treatment (the first and second problems discussed
above) may be paid, whilst no symptomatic improvement is experienced. The converse also applies. For example, there is evidence to
suggest that the scope for spontaneous recovery for people suffering
from major depression is considerable. Patients in placebo groups of
controlled trials receiving no treatment demonstrate a major improvement after four weeks of between 40 and 60 per cent (Freemantle *et
al.*, 1993). These individuals improved without being exposed to the
iatrogenic risks entailed in the treatment condition. 'Spontaneous' improvement from emotional problems may be a misleading misnomer
as it implies a change which is in some sense remarkable or even
mysterious. In fact, people untreated by a medical intervention may
utilise lay relationships to ameliorate their distress. People in control
groups continue to have relationships, and some of these may be benign
and supportive.

(6) Randomised controlled trials (efficacy studies) which are not
'pragmatic trials,' are methodologically pure but are also *unrepresen-
tative of actual practice*. In efficacy studies 'manual-driven' standardised
treatments are studied as single interventions with atypical patient populations and specifiable symptoms are ranked before and after treatment
(or control). Drop-outs are eliminated as a contaminating variable. In
actual services, people drop in and out of treatment. They often have
complex rather than single problems. They may often be receiving more
than one treatment concurrently and 'treatment fidelity' (the compliance
of the therapist, not the patient with treatment delivery) may vary. Thus
a different literature (not the 'gold standard' of efficacy studies) about
in situ treatment is required to understand how treatment works in
actual clinical settings. This leads us to our next question.

What evidence is there that actual services engender cost-effective treatments?

'Effectiveness' refers to the utility of interventions; put simply, do they work or do they do what we expect from them? 'Efficiency' refers to cost-effectiveness. If several interventions are equally effective then the most efficient one would be the cheapest. An expensive technique may be clinically effective in an individual case but a health economist might consider the cost to be too high for the health gain produced in a population or when compared to a cheaper but less effective alternative. The arguments about the merits of different types of anti-depressants highlight this (Freemantle and Maynard, 1994). The new anti-depressants (SSRIs) are clinically effective and (their advocates argue) are more cost-effective because they do not lead to the accident rates associated with the old tricyclic drugs. The latter create greater sedation effects. However, the advocates of the old drugs point out that their substantial cheapness makes them a better buy, as they are just as clinically effective as the new drugs. Freemantle and Maynard are sceptical about the claims made on both sides and consider that a rational comparison of the drugs is made difficult by the research on the SSRIs being sponsored by their commercial producers.

For health economists, 'efficiency' relates not just to the optimal treatment, in terms of clinical outcome, but the maximum social/health benefit of that treatment within the constraints of resource allocation. Le Grand and Robinson (1981) have defined efficiency as 'that output at which the excess of benefits over costs, called the net benefit, is largest'. This involves three associated concepts: benefits to consumers, the costs of production, and an efficient level of output. Efficiency, then, needs to take account of *costs* as well as the benefits of health care. For example, in relation to the treatment of schizophrenia, a number of economic evaluation studies have attempted to show that Clozapine (a new anti-psychotic drug) is cost-effective for use in relation to so-called 'treatment-resistant' patients. Despite the cost entailed in monitoring recipients for the known side-effect of agranulocytosis (a potentially fatal blood disorder), it is claimed that Clozapine performs well in comparison with other 'anti-psychotic' drugs. Its advocates claim that it reduces hospital admissions for a particularly expensive group of patients by enhancing both social functioning and quality of life.

Returning, then, to the methodological challenge about effective services, each local service would need its own tailored audit mechanisms to check the following:

1   Do professionals actually utilise evidence from efficacy studies, and
    do they put evidence into practice?
2   Do users report advantages and disadvantages: do they feel better
    after service contact?
3   Does cost (not clinical) effectiveness guide professional practice
    and service organisation?

Currently we know much less about this information because it is either
not generated systematically in all localities or it is produced but not
disseminated. Dissemination is impeded by criteria operating in professional journals about suitability for publication. Large efficacy studies
readily fit these publication criteria, whereas small pieces of local audit
work do not. Thus the information about the state of *actual services*
can only be accessed, in the main, via a 'grey literature' of disparate
pieces of local work of variable availability and varying methodology
accumulating in research reports.

Do services offer treatments on an equitable basis?

Equity is a moral and political issue and is not just about effectiveness. A service may be ineffective but people may wish to have free
and ready access to it, independent of their ability to pay. The
expressed need for equitable access to mental health interventions
is very uneven. For example, users complain of lacking choice and not
having ready access to talking treatments, or 24-hour help. At the same
time, as we will see later, the fact that some social groups are overrepresented in psychiatric populations is a cause for concern, not celebration.
   Three common definitions of equity are used in a health care context:

(a) a minimum standard of care for all of those in need;
(b) equal treatment for equal need;
(c) equality of access.

In relation to people with mental health problems, how these definitions of equity are put into operation will depend on who is doing the
defining. The notion of need is likely to differ according to whether it
is defined by purchasers, mental health professionals or users. For
example, in relation to point (c), the expressed need of a person to be
referred to a counsellor may not accord with the opinion of a psychiatrist, if that person's problem is not viewed as severe enough to

constitute 'clinical depression'. A minimum standard of care relates to whether or not someone in acute distress is offered *some* sort of help, such as admission to hospital. The second notion of equity above refers to the extent to which a type of treatment or facility is made available to people with the same or similar difficulties. An example is in relation to the availability of therapeutic communities. Not all those deemed to have a personality disorder by psychiatrists will have the option of such a treatment regime.

Huxley (1990), in his overview of the literature on effectiveness, notes that the notion of a comprehensive service appears in three senses:

• comprehensive response to the mental health needs of a population
• comprehensive provision of services
• comprehensive care of the individual client's needs.

These distinctions are important in relation to service evaluation because they are practical proxy measures of equitable service delivery which are not always commensurable. For example, it is possible for those in contact with services to be dealt with successfully in line with the third version above. At the same time in that locality there could be unmet need in the population (a failure by the first criterion). Patmore and Weaver (1991, 4) interpret a 'comprehensive' service as being one which 'can address, as required, needs for money and housing, care for physical illness, leisure and social life, occupation, psychiatric medication, emergency support, liaison with family and help with daily living skills'. Thus their definition is focused on the individual client (Huxley's third version above). (The arguments about whether and how individual intensive case management works in the community were debated in Chapter 9 in relation to British and North American models of service organisation.)

Do Services Improve the Quality of Life of Patients?

In addition to providing a cost-effective and equitable service, the notion of acceptability is also an emerging consideration. Acceptability is implicit in the concepts of effectiveness and efficiency: any attempt to measure benefits of treatments requires information as to the value placed on it in terms of improvements in mental health by those in receipt of service delivery. As we saw in the last chapter, this reflects the increasing credence being given to the expressed needs of service users. A good example is the controversy about the use of ECT. Psychiatrists argue that it is a useful and legitimate treatment option and that it is clinically effective. By contrast, users find it frightening and often unacceptable (Rogers and Pilgrim, 1994). (MIND are currently campaigning to reduce its use in general psychiatry.)

Twenty years ago the notion that treatments should be acceptable to their recipients was rarely, if ever, heard; now it is commonplace. Quality of life has two components in relation to mental health service contact. The first refers to consumer satisfaction (whether services respond to expressed need and whether they are acceptable and accessible to recipients). The second is whether the patient's general citizenship is enhanced or diminished by service contact. These are different and may contradict one another at times. Patients may be satisfied with their treatment but the stigmatising impact of service contact may reduce their job prospects.

The overall problem of defining both service quality and need satisfaction is summarised succinctly here by Beazley (1994):

> Legal definitions of need are fairly narrow and mainly refer to needs for particular services . . . rather than the wider view about the need for social care based on ideas about quality of life. The ability of a service to 'satisfy' a need is difficult to assess, as there are few examples of studies or effective systems yet in operation which draw directly on the opinions of service users.

One priority for those commissioning and running services is to ensure that they are acceptable to those who use them. The research on this topic to date tends to damn inpatient provision. The results of a national survey conducted by us for National MIND (Rogers, Pilgrim and Lacey, 1993) showed that users often found inpatient services to be humiliating and the environment depressing and felt a loss of citizenship. Some of the sample, including informal patients, reported coercion and brutality from staff. Outpatient services were criticised for long waiting times, short consultation times, and inconsistent medical staffing, although some clients welcomed the access to psychiatrists and viewed the service in preventive terms.

Day care centres, still often linked to hospital sites, were seen as being inaccessible and extensions of the hospital regimen, with a lack of meaningful activity and continuing sense of coercion being commented on. Opening times were seen as inflexible. Clients enjoyed contact with other users and found staff to be more helpful than their hospital counterparts. Many clients who valued day care centres were concerned about cutbacks in services, which is at odds with the prioritising of non-inpatient services.

A spate of studies point clearly to the conclusion that patients prefer to be treated outside hospital. Rogers, Pilgrim and Lacey (1993) found that the further services are from hospital the more they are appreciated by service-users. McIntyre, Farrell and David (1989) found that 'the thing that inpatients most like about being in hospital is their ability to leave'. Marks (1992) found that the relatives of patients also prefer community care to hospital care. Other studies also indicate that community-based treatment is not only preferred but it is also a more cost-effective method of care. One particular disadvantage of service contact is that admission to hospital jeopardises housing tenure (Bean and Mounser, 1995).

Dean and Gadd (1990) investigated the outcome of UK community treatment of severe acute psychiatric illnesses that were traditionally treated in hospital. They found that home treatment was a feasible option for most patients and that success of home treatment could be improved by a locally-based mental health resource centre, a 24-hour on-call service, an open referral system, and an active follow-up policy. Given that what patients most like about hospital is their ability to leave (McIntyre, Farrell and David, 1989), that hospital ward regimes are 'non-therapeutic' (Sainsbury Centre, 1998) and that hospital stays are correlated negatively with user satisfaction with service quality (Clarkson and McCrone, 1998), it would seem that a minimal building block of enhanced quality of life is to keep people out of hospital.

Whilst the preference for community, rather than hospital-based, care is a consistent signal from research on users' views, the same research also highlights the problem of defining need satisfaction by service preference alone. Put simply, people with mental health problems are not just people who act oddly and/or experience distress: they are also devalued individuals with precarious rights of citizenship. Even if services were organised less and less on an inpatient basis, this would not in itself solve wider problems of social marginalisation and exclusion.

There are wide-ranging practical problems which affect people with mental health problems. Rogers, Pilgrim and Lacey (1993) found that the issues of greatest concern were money, accommodation, a need for employment or occupation, as well as services and their staff. They also established that users' employment prospects were severely and irreversibly damaged as a result of having been a psychiatric patient. Many users find it very difficult to live on the money available to them and many are poorly informed about their rights to loans, grants, allowances and benefits (Hogman and Melzer, 1992). Choice of accommodation is often very limited for many users returning to the community, with a fair number ultimately spending time in group homes, hostels or other emergency housing.

An important point made by Clarkson and McCrone (1998) is that it is very difficult to interpret the meaning of mental health service users reporting poor quality of life. Is it that the underlying reasons for the latter (poverty, restricted social networks, stigma, poor education and employment) are so profound and pervasive that disappointment with services reflects an incorrigible state of poor self-esteem and alienation about everything in the patient's world? Under these circumstances service users may be suffering a deep-seated impoverishment and disempowerment created by their social conditions, but they attribute the state to service inadequacies.

Given that subjective reports of quality of life and other professionally-defined indices of successful psychiatric rehabilitation are applied in community settings (Oliver *et al.*, 1996) it is difficult to disaggregate service factors from others impinging on the patient. Maybe quality of life is overdetermined by extra-service factors. Alternatively, services may fail to reverse alienation, and might even compound pre-existing socially created difficulties. Either interpretation still leaves services lacking. They are either having no impact on quality of life in the face of wider negative social factors or they are making matters worse. The latter possibility is more likely in relation to those patients who have services imposed upon them compulsorily, bringing us to our next point.

Do Services Effectively Control Risky Behaviour?

We noted at the start of this chapter that whether it is conceded or not, mental health services are in the business, partially at least, of coercive social control. In this section we consider not *whether* mental health professionals are in the business of coercive control but *when* they are, do they act effectively? That is, in actual services are mental health professionals effective at reducing the probability of harm to self and others in those deemed to have mental health problems? Our response to this question will be dealt with under two headings.

Self-harm

A difficulty in estimating the impact of mental health services on self-harm is that the latter concept includes many elements. For example, people may indulge in many activities which jeopardise their quality of life, their longevity or their health. Two good examples of this are cigarette smoking and driving fast. Some risky roles are even socially valued (mountaineers, astronauts and racing car drivers.) As Szasz (1963) noted, it is not acting dangerously *per se* that is the issue but the *way* in which one is dangerous. Despite this complexity, legislation is passed about mental health which glibly allows others to pass judgement and take action about the control of risky behaviour. Also, the availability of dangerous *means* may remain highly unregulated, whilst very specific sanctions are imposed on dangerous *individuals*. A good example of this contradiction is that in the USA mental health law is readily invoked to control suicidal intent or parasuicidal action but lax gun laws give people easy access to lethal means. In this country the same is true but in relation to paracetamol retail. Whilst we know that people with psychiatric diagnoses (especially schizophrenia and depression) have higher rates of suicide than the general population, it is not clear currently whether services are effective in reducing or preventing suicide, once the risk of self-harm is detected. This point is reinforced by the high base rate of suicide *in acute inpatient units* where surveillance is maximised.

Harm to others

Despite prejudicial reporting in the mass media and biased political decision-making in its wake (Dobson, 1998), we do have a reasonably clear understanding about the degree of dangerous threat which psychiatric patients pose to others. Taken as whole population, people with mental health problems, even those who have had inpatient stays, are actually less dangerous than their non-mentally ill neighbours. However, within this total population some patients are predictably violent. Risk factors which raise the probability of violence include the following.

1   The use of illicit drugs and/or alcohol. Discharged patients who abuse street drugs and alcohol are substantially at risk of assaulting others. It is also important to note here that drug and alcohol use *alone* predict violence. However, the concurrence of psychosis and substance abuse interact to produce a greater risk of violence.

2   Those patients with command hallucinations (voices telling them to harm others) and delusions with hostile content (fear of aggression from perceived enemies or hostile conspirators) are more likely to harm others than those with other symptoms.

3   Those with a diagnosis of anti-social personality disorder (ASP) are dangerous. This is the most predictable correlated predictive factor, albeit because of circular reasoning. The diagnosis accrues from past anti-social acts. Given that past behaviour is the best predictor of future behaviour, it is not surprising that arsonists or murderers with a psychiatric label of personality disorder may well repeat their actions. Perpetrators of both sexual and non-sexual violence receive the ASP label in secure psychiatric facilities.

Having indicated these three main points about risk in psychiatric populations, it is equally important to note that most patients are not violent
and that most violence in society is not committed by patients. Psychiatric
diagnosis *per se* is not a good predictor of violence whereas gender
(male) and age (young) are (with or without a diagnosis). Moreover,
as has already been noted, the best predictor of violence in individuals
is past violence (independent of their mental state). This picture has
led those studying mental disorder and violence to emphasise that we
can become preoccupied with clinical variables (diagnosis, symptoms,
etc.) and ignore more general actuarial and biographical factors (of
gender, age, class and criminality: see Monahan and Steadman, 1994).

   In the light of this general picture, how do services fare in controlling dangerousness? One answer to this question lies in the *inherent
success* of preventative detention. That is, where mental health services lock up those with risky behaviour, then they are for the duration
keeping potential assailants out of contact with potential victims in
community settings. However, they are also concentrating risky behaviour
in psychiatric settings (acute inpatient units, Regional Secure Units
and Special Hospitals). Not surprisingly, there is evidence of high rates
of assault in these settings. A more difficult question to answer is whether
the *interventions* which occur in such services are effective at reducing dangerousness post-discharge. The tendency of those deemed to be
seriously dangerous to spend long periods of time in conditions of
psychiatric detention could point to a slow rate of discharge because
of the poor success of interventions. An alternative explanation is that
preventative detention (custodialism) becomes the main cultural motif
of inpatient services. If detention becomes an aim in itself and patients
receive little corrective attention for their violent propensities, then it

is not surprising that discharge is slow. The complaint of lack of thera-peutic activity in psychiatric facilities goes back to the Victorian asylums. Recent inquiries and site visits suggest that very little has changed in acute units (Sainsbury Centre, 1998) and in secure hospitals (Fallon Inquiry, 1998).

Quality Assurance

The quality assurance literature suggests that certain recurring criteria may be used to audit mental health services and appraise whether or not they are providing value for money. It is common now to use six memorable criteria about service quality: the three As and the three Es. These refer to access, acceptability, appropriateness, equity, effec-tiveness and efficiency. These six criteria can then be set against three dimensions of services: structure, process and outcome (SPO). Struc-tural factors refer to *what* is provided (buildings, personnel, beds, skill mix of staff). Structure is also about volume (how many staff, etc.) and so is a good measure of service investment. Process by contrast is about *how* a service is delivered: the nature of the relationships in-volved (impersonal, friendly, benign, harsh, respectful, cursory, protracted, etc.). Outcome refers to some measure of success (observed improve-ments in presenting problems, client reports of satisfaction, cheapest way to achieve a result, etc.).

A service may boast good outcomes in terms of accessibility but may be delivering ineffective treatments (or vice versa). Also the SPO dimensions highlight that stakeholders focus on different elements of the services. For example, professionals often emphasise the need for *more volume*, such as more posts for their own discipline, or more beds for their local service. This is why politicians have become adept at separating the special pleading of health service tribalism (a request to boost structure) from whether or not it will lead to improved ser-vice outcomes. Users and their significant others, like politicians, are more interested in outcomes, especially ones of acceptability and ac-cessibility. They are not always in a position to judge whether an intervention is appropriate, effective or efficient and as individuals they may be little concerned with whether the service is equitable. Some argue that the most important form of understanding is about the P–O link: that is, how do professionals need to deliver services in order to generate successful outcomes (Brugha and Lindsay, 1996).

Women, Men and Service Contact

Concerns about the discrimination against and oppression of, female patients culminated in the National MIND campaign concerning women and mental health, which is in progress. An extensive recent review of services for women (Williams *et al.*, 1993) highlights a number of discriminatory processes. Services are prone to:

- misdiagnose women's distress
- fail to help women deal with the causes of their problems
- mistreat women's distress by using inappropriate medication and ECT, and by inappropriately admitting them to hospital
- be unsafe for women

Williams *et al.* argue that distressed women who approach the mental health service are often automatically assumed to have biological or biochemical problems or inter-personal difficulties, which cause them to be mentally ill. They believe that what actually underlies women's distress is their experience of social inequality on a daily basis. Poverty, much more common amongst women than men, is associated with psychological distress (Bruce, Takeuchi and Keaf, 1991). This situation is exacerbated when experienced in combination with the stress of caring for children and other dependents, which is an exacting experience in itself. Childbirth is estimated to be associated with depression in 10–30 per cent of cases (Nicolson, 1989), and domestic violence is similarly linked to long-term mental health problems. Williams *et al.* (1993) identify older women, homeless women, lesbian women and black and ethnic minority women as particular groups who are vulnerable to disadvantage and discrimination.

Older women are more likely to receive psychotropic drugs and less likely to be offered talking treatments than any other group (Catalan, Gath and Bond, 1988). Since they are the group that is most at risk from side-effects of drugs (Grohmann *et al.*, 1989), this is of significant concern. As 60 per cent of women over the age of 65 live below the official poverty line (Titley, Watson and Williams, 1992), the links between poverty and mental distress are of particular relevance to them.

Williams *et al.* (1993) cite research which suggests that homeless women are more likely than homeless men to report mental health problems or that they have been hospitalised in the past (Crystel, Ladner and Towber, 1986; Hagen, 1990). They also note that homelessness is on the increase amongst older people, especially women. There is much evidence which links sexual and physical abuse to mental distress, and Akilu (1991) found that such abuse can also be related to women becoming homeless.

Martin and Lyon (1984) and Rothblum (1990) argue that lesbian women are at a particular disadvantage due to mental health service providers assuming that all patients are heterosexual. They also argue that homophobia in services can cause additional stress and is associated with the idea that mental health problems stem from these patients' particular sexual orientation and lifestyle. (These pressures within the mental health system may well apply to homosexual men.)

The black and ethnic minority communities are particularly poorly served by the mental health service. Whilst many of the issues relating to this point will be discussed in the next section, it is important to emphasise that much of the literature fails to accentuate or differentiate the particular needs of black and ethnic women as opposed to black and ethnic minority men. One would surmise that the combined effects of gender and race place a double burden upon these women. However, the interaction between gender and race is complex. For example, whereas Irish women appear to suffer more mental health problems than their male equivalents, the reverse is true of Afro-Caribbean people (see next section).

A number of studies conducted in psychiatric hospitals have found that a significant proportion of female patients (figures ranged from 46 to 72 per cent) have previously experienced abuse (Carmen, Ricker and Mills, 1984; Bryers *et al.*, 1987; Herman, Perrey and vander Kolk, 1989). These findings coincide with the conclusions of community studies of women using psychiatric services or attending women's projects (Rose, Peabody and Stratigeas, 1991; Mills, 1992). Williams *et al.* (1993) suggest that abuse is strongly linked with high service use. Women who have been abused are prescribed more medication, are admitted to hospital for longer periods of time and whilst in hospital are more likely to spend time in seclusion than women who have not experienced abuse. A history of sexual or physical abuse is also associated with depression, eating difficulties and heightened rates of self-harm and suicidal thoughts and attempts. Abuse can be experienced whilst patients are using mental health services, whether it be inflicted by staff, other patients or therapists (Nilbert, Cooper and Crossmaker, 1989; Edwards and Fasal, 1992; Garrett, 1992).

These examples of discrimination and oppression experienced by female psychiatric patients can be considered against a different set of problems for male patients. Men's behaviour is more frequently recognised as dangerous than is women's, and this may have as much to do with stereotypical expectations as it does with fact. Women's behaviour is often associated with private, self-damaging acts, with aggression being directed inwards and leading to self-mutilation, depression and eating disorders. Men's behaviour has been associated more with public anti-social acts such as drunken, aggressive behaviour and violent and/or sexual offences. As a result, men are more likely to be labelled as criminally deviant than are women. Therefore, women are seen stereo-typically as being a danger to themselves, whilst men are seen stereotypically as being a danger to others; consequently within psychiatry men are more likely to have labels which refer to and incorporate the threat of their behaviour.

Women are more likely to be dealt with in primary health care settings at the 'soft' end of psychiatry, whilst men are more likely to be dealt with at that 'harsh' end, particularly at the interface between psychiatry and the criminal justice system. In 'special hospitals', it is men who are overrepresented, despite the fact that in some instances they have not been convicted of a criminal offence. Men are subject to removal more frequently than women under Section 136 of the Mental Health Act, and the police use handcuffs and detention cells more frequently for men than women in these circumstances (Rogers, 1990). Thus although feminist researchers have accurately identified particular risks for women in relation to service contact, men also suffer risks, but these are of a different type.

Race, Ethnicity and Service Contact

Compared to other groups in the population, Afro-Caribbean (and Irish) people are overrepresented in psychiatric admissions to hospitals. However, precise data on this is not always available since ethnic monitoring does not always take place consistently across health and social services. Afro-Caribbean people are much more likely than white people to make contact with psychiatry via the police, courts and prison system. They are detained under Section 136 of the 1983 Mental Health Act at two-and-a-half times the rate of whites living in the same locality, and they tend to be young and male (Bean *et al.*, 1991). McGovern and Cope (1987) and Cope (1989) found that migrant and British-born second-generation Afro-Caribbean men were found to be twenty-nine times more likely than white males to be referred under Part III of the

Mental Health Act, which makes provision for dealing with patients involved in criminal proceedings or serving a prison sentence.

A study of people discharged from Special Hospitals found that there were higher proportions of 'non-whites' than would be expected from the general population and that the 'non-white' group had committed less serious offences prior to admission (Norris, 1984). Browne (1990) found that black defendants were less likely to be granted bail and more likely to receive court orders involving compulsory psychiatric treatment than their white counterparts. In contrast to this, there is evidence that black people are underrepresented in outpatient and self-referred services (Littlewood and Cross, 1980), and are less likely than other groups to be referred by general practitioners (Hitch and Clegg, 1980).

There are a number of theories as to why black people are overrepresented in psychiatric statistics. Some psychiatrists argue that it is simply a reflection of a greater incidence of severe mental illness in black people (Cope, 1989). By contrast, Francis (1989) views it as an indication of the way in which psychiatry forms part of a larger social control apparatus which regulates and oversees the lives of black people. Since black people, particularly young black men, are overrepresented in all parts of the criminal justice system, the 'criminalisation' and 'medicalisation' of black people may be closely connected processes.

This thesis is strengthened when we look at the type of service contact that black people have. Whilst most people enter psychiatric facilities informally, the chances that Afro-Caribbean people will do so are much smaller. Cope (1989) found that 20–30 per cent of Afro-Caribbean patients were detained involuntarily, compared with 8 per cent of the total compulsory admissions to the hospital system during the 1980s. Young Afro-Caribbean migrants were found to be admitted at 17 times the community rate for compulsory admissions and at 25 times the community rate for admissions via the criminal justice system (Cope, 1989).

Afro-Caribbean people are overrepresented in locked wards and secure units (Bolton, 1984; Jones and Berry, 1986) and ECT is overused in the treatment of Afro-Caribbean and Asian patients (Littlewood and Cross, 1980; Shaikh, 1985). Furthermore, black patients are more likely to receive major tranquillisers and intra-muscular medication (Littlewood and Cross, 1980); be seen by junior medical staff (Littlewood and Cross, 1980); and receive higher levels of medication over time (Chen, Harrison and Standen, 1991). Because of this coercive emphasis, it is not surprising that black people may avoid contact with statutory services and favour contact with black organisations in the voluntary sector

(Goldberg *et al.*, 1993). Thus it would seem that statutory mental health services are not merely discriminatory in relation to black people but that they are not learning currently from good practice in the voluntary sector.

The alienation of the black community from statutory mental health services was recognised by the NHS Executive Mental Health Task Force (DH, 1994b) and its messages have been endorsed by John Bowis, junior Health Minister (DH, 1994d). The Task Force conclusions included that mental health service purchasers and providers should:

* develop the role of the black non-statutory sector
* improve consultation and communication to bring black communities, including users and carers, into the planning structure
* develop closer working relationships with local community fora
* acknowledge the work and experience of black professionals in statutory organisations
* build independent advocacy into service monitoring
* include culturally appropriate methods of assessment and intervention

Discussion

The concerns expressed by black groups and feminist researchers about the overrepresentation of black people and women in psychiatric facilities raise an important point about mental health services. Whereas equity of access to the NHS is politically valued in relation to physical health problems, the excessive contact by some social groups is considered to be problematic in relation to mental health services.

There are four possible explanations for this contradiction, which are not mutually exclusive. First, especially in relation to compulsory admission to hospital, service contact is often not about the expressed needs of patients being met but is about the resolution of social crises in public or domestic settings. It is difficult to determine who is the central client of psychiatry: the indentified patient or others affected by their behaviour? Second, psychiatric services are linked to the old lunatic asylum and have had an unbroken history of stigma. Third, psychiatric treatments (not just containment) are sometimes experienced as personally distressing, socially disabling or oppressive. Fourth, as part of a wider system of social control, psychiatry has become one of several sites for the manifestation of institutionalised racism and sexism in society. Taking these points together, it is not surprising that service contact is often seen by current and prospective users not as a right to be enjoyed but as an imposition to be suffered or endured. This may account for why politicised service-users often describe themselves as 'survivors' of the psychiatric system.

Thus, the effectiveness of mental health services remains problematic for a number of reasons which are a product of the separate domains we have highlighted earlier in this chapter *and* as a result of them coming into conflict. We can think of two broad sources of inefficiency. The first is about *professional limitations*, some of which mental health workers are responsible for and others not. As we noted earlier, professionals are not always efficient in their therapeutic aspirations. Not all therapies work all the time for all clients. Not all therapists act with personal integrity and they may fail to show treatment fidelity. Similarly, risk prediction and management is still more of an art than a science, given the problems of making accurate predictions in open systems. As for quality of life, this is often outside the control of professionals as it is bound up with factors such as material resources, social networks and labour market disadvantage.

Apart from professional inefficiency there are also *service contradictions*. If mental health services were *only* in the business of reducing the symptoms of madness and distress, this would be difficult enough, but it would made easier if professionals did not have to concern themselves with considerations of risk management and life quality. (A good case example of therapeutic purism excluding wider considerations is offered by Barron (1988) when describing a therapeutic community which became hopelessly dysfunctional.) Similarly, risk management would be made much easier if mental health services *only* had to focus on risk minimisation; they would lock many people up for very long periods of time in order to prevent them harming themselves or others. But to do this would be profoundly socially disabling and would generally create, not reduce, distress in patients. Given that personal liberty is such a fundamental precondition and feature of citizenship, *only* working to enhance quality of life might jeopardise symptom reduction in some and would certainly raise the probability of risky behaviour in others. A good example of the tension here is in relation to assertive outreach. This seems to be highly effective at reducing psychotic symptomatology but it is intrusive and thus may undermine citizenship.

In this light, mental health services and those who work in them are subject to a 'cruciform effect' (Gowler and Legge, 1980). That is, which ever way they twist and turn to find a new, more comfortable compromise between the three functions described, new painful outcomes may occur as each solution breeds a new problem. Efficiency at one function regularly creates inefficiency in, or contradicts, another. This profoundly pessimistic conclusion about mental health services can only be tempered if professionals are honest and humble (Pilgrim, 1998). If treatment efficiency, optimal risk management and improved quality of life are problematic to ensure separately and together, then professionals need to be honest about this struggle. Honesty is also implied about the notion of 'mental health care'. This safe catch-all category disguises the conflict between treatment and control. The concerns expressed about race and gender above suggest that there has to be an honest acknowledgement that mental health services are, in part at least, one wing of a repressive State apparatus or an important element in the moral regulation of a social order.

Having concluded that mental health services can never be all things to all people, the residual implication for effectiveness is that the State has to ensure that the resources are present for staff to maximise their efficiency in treatment and risk management, and for service-users to maximise their quality of life. These resources are partly material (adequately financed services, available choice of accommodation, labour market opportunities and income maintenance). They are also partly political, since professionals need to be supported doing a difficult job but should also be accountable and transparent in their functioning. Equally, users need to be supported to assert their individual and collective rights. Even if resource enhancement were to be ensured by the State, mental health services would still remain riven with contradictions and so notions of service effectiveness would require clear conceptual analysis.

12

Past, Present and Future

In Chapter 4 a number of factors were considered about British mental health policy in the late twentieth century. This chapter moves to an appraisal of the implications of these factors for the coming years. To start this process we return to the three-tier analytical framework, introduced at the start of the book (Pilgrim and Rogers, 1999). Macro, meso and micro factors will be sub-headings for the appraisal and tentative predictions.

Macro Factors

These represent the enduring, if cyclical, issues about mental abnormality and its societal response. In one sense little has changed in relation to the historical picture, dating back to ancient Greece and Rome, about madness. The latter was associated with violence and aimless wandering. It is evident still today that policy responses are in large part about the control of risky behaviour and the containment of those transgressing rules and creating social crises. What is only of recent historical relevance (the last two hundred years) is that the state should offer a centralised or standardised set of solutions to the social problems of risk and residence associated with madness, whether these include the asylum system or acute hospitalisation plus community care to support those with enduring problems when not in crisis. What has only been of real relevance for less than a hundred years are aspects of mental abnormality which lie outside madness, such as ordinary distress, phobias, general anxiety states, depression, personality problems. It is only in the last 50 years that any notion of positive mental health has been considered as a policy matter.

Thus, from a macro perspective, there are accumulating layers of policy over time. In the future, therefore, the *aggregate* of these issues about madness, distress and well-being will be addressed in some way or other by policy-makers. Moreover, this aggregate picture is, for the foreseeable future, going to be linked to the notion of *services*. It is important to remember that this notion is peculiarly modern. In the eighteenth century there were madhouses. In the nineteenth we had asylums. Now we have mental health services. When we think of mental health policy, the relatively short time frame of this service discourse needs to be borne in mind.

Moving from time to space, a question remains about whether or not a narrow convergence is evident internationally about mental health policy. Psychiatric knowledge remains embedded in the international classification system preferred by the World Health Organisation (currently ICD10). This is important because it is used by many countries as an epidemiological basis for estimating the prevalence of mental disorders in a nation-state and allocating resources in response. It is the basis for the training of psychiatrists and psychiatric nurses and is used in diagnostic procedures in courts of law. However, ICD10 competes with another classification system (DSM-IV) produced by the American Psychiatric Association. ICD10 was roughly based on DSM-II and DSM-IV diverges from its predecessor in an important respect. DSM-II and ICD10 follow old classification contours which divided groups of patients who were diagnosed as suffering from some version of psychosis, neurosis or personality disorder. DSM-IV moved from this traditional categorical approach to one elaborated by an axial approach. In Britain *both* systems operate in parallel, which clouds decision-making for policy-makers based upon a medical model.

More generally in health policy, services are planned and their efficiency evaluated in relation to Diagnostic Related Groups (DRGs). This is problematic in Britain if DSM-IV and ICD10 are in competition for pre-eminent legitimacy (which they are). A transhistorical problem that also remains unresolved in both systems is that of aetiology. Most psychiatric disorders are defined functionally (i.e., by symptoms), and have no clear biological markers (signs). Even though aetiological speculation remains heavily biologically oriented, causes remain contested, as do their status, therefore, as proper diseases. Organic psychoses, temporal lobe epilepsy and dementia are neurological conditions dealt with less often by mental health services than depression, anxiety and the functional psychoses. Even in older people depression is a much commoner diagnosis than dementia. This leaves the bulk of psychiatric epidemiology weak in comparison to medical epidemiology. The latter in its exact or pure form should offer policy-makers a formula to map out not just the distribution of DRGs but also their *likely causes*. Psychiatric epidemiology, whichever classificatory system it uses, cannot offer the latter information for the great bulk of cases. Thus, a recurring problem for policy-makers in coming years is going to be its reliance on psychiatric epidemiological data for its decision-making. However, the limits of a DRG approach are now being recognised by government, with risk, vulnerability and need displacing diagnosis in practice guidance (DH, 1999).

Whether or not dubious DRGs are used in policy formation, the question about containing and controlling madness remain. As a consequence, there are indications that globally there has been a convergence in mental health policy across a variety of nations about the control of behaviour which offends societal norms. Some countries are more liberal and others more authoritarian about this focus, but the question of the threat posed to society by mad behaviour remains central across nations.

A related convergence is that of the organisation and financing of mental health services. For example, the optimal use of limited budgets for mental health services has led to North American policy analysts noting that the USA and Britain in the early 1990s were offering fragmented services with splits between primary and secondary care, in terms of budgetary control and management. This led to some successful experiments in Philadelphia, Utah and Oregon to unify mental health services to maximise their efficiency and to overcome the problems of fragmentation (Hadley and Goldman, 1995). The latter authors note that the political arrangements in Britain during the last term of prolonged Conservative government created the same problems of fragmentation as in the USA, in the wake of the 1990 NHS and Community Care Act. The currently emerging solution in Britain, like the American experiments, is of implementing unitary mental health trusts and of pooling NHS and social service budgets. Thus a convergence can be seen over the past ten years between the USA and Britain about the reversal of inefficient, fragmented mental health services. The finer details of the current British scene will now be examined.

Meso Factors

These are the ones which fit into a traditional social administrative framework about policy formation and implementation: that is, national government legislation and guidance about mental health. At the time of writing, mental health services are being uncoupled from the determinants and constraints of legislation in the early 1990s, especially the 1990 NHS and Community Care Act. In addition, the extant mental legislation (the 1983 Mental Health Act) will probably be displaced by a new law. The most significant shift is in relation to government ideology. The Conservative administration prior to 1997 attempted to use a bureaucratic mechanism (managerialism) in combination with a non-bureaucratic mechanism (the 'internal market') to raise the efficiency of the health and social services.

In contrast to this pre-1997 picture, we now have a set of possibilities being created by a Labour government coming to the end of its first term. It is relevant to consider here a set of interlocking pieces of policy documentation. In particular, the following will be discussed: *A First Class Service* (DH, 1998a); the *National Service Framework for Mental Health*; *Health Outcome Indicators for Mental Illness*; and the scoping exercise about new mental health legislation alongside the government's Green Paper on the topic, *Reform of the Mental Health Act 1983*.

A First Class Service: *the 'driver' of clinical governance*

Clinical governance is a central part of current government thinking about improving standards in the NHS. It emphasises quality improvements and local corporate professional responsibility for these improvements. Consequently it brings together and thus supersedes two distinct traditional power bases in the NHS of clinicians and general managers. Moreover, whereas the notion of 'clinician' was associated in the past with medical practitioners, the new emphasis on collective professional responsibility entails multi-disciplinarity. Multi-disciplinary groups of practitioners are expected to take responsibility for clinical governance in their part of the service (for our purposes here, specialist mental health services or mental health care within primary care). In the case of specialist services, the Chief Executive of NHS Trusts or the Chief Officers of PCGs are held responsible for delivering clinical governance and will be under scrutiny from the NHSE and the Commission for Health Improvement. Thus the political strategy of clinical governance aims at enforcing local responsibility for service quality and it establishes lines of accountability about this responsibility.

In *A First Class Service* (DH, 1998a) a tripartite rationale was announced. This consisted of a standard-setting system (the National Institute of Clinical Excellence and National Service Frameworks), a delivery system (clinical governance) and a monitoring system (the Commission for Health Improvement, the National Performance Assessment Framework and the National Survey of Patients). Clinical governance is defined in *A First Class Service* as 'a framework through which NHS organisations are accountable for continuously improving the quality of their services and safeguarding high standards of care by creating an environment in which excellence in clinical care will flourish'. It consists of five main overlapping activities which were present under the previous managerial emphasis within the NHS during the 1980s and early 1990s (though less obviously in primary care than in specialist care), as detailed below.

1   The first and overarching activity is about *quality improvement* which is understood, minimally, to be about ensuring that services are increasingly cost-effective and accessible. Broader quality frameworks also include other criteria such as appropriateness, acceptability and equity, although it might be argued that these additional criteria could be subsumed under the minimal two of effectiveness and accessibility (Buetow and Roland, 1999: see Chapter 11 above). Quality improvement includes innovations and initiatives to change service for the better using existing evidence about best practice. It also subsumes the next activity.

2   A second and more focused activity is about raising the performance in one or a few specified clinical areas in a locality. This involves identifying the gap, if any, between what a service tries to deliver (according to stated intentions such as operational policies) and what it actually delivers. This is *clinical audit*, entailing collecting information to identify deviations from good practice and then setting up corrective action to alter the service for the better (the 'audit cycle').

3   The third activity is about ensuring that interventions deployed in a service are *effective* according to research evidence (known as 'evidence-based practice' or sometimes 'evidence-based medicine').

4   The fourth activity is about *risk assessment and management*, again in accordance with evidence. In mental health services this has mainly been associated with minimising risky client behaviour (self-harm, self-neglect and harm to others). However, it shades over into questions of clinical effectiveness when risk of services and their interventions *to* clients (iatrogenic risk) is considered (Pilgrim and Rogers, 1998: see below).

5   A fifth service feature is then prescribed by government: a workforce

trained in the skills and evidence required to deliver the four activities in each locality. This activity is known as *continuous professional development*. Strictly, this is not envisaged by government as being an element of clinical governance but it is is seen as underpinning quality improvement.

At the time of writing, it is not possible to predict the precise impact of clinical governance (see Chapter 5), although some general points can be made. As a quality improvement strategy, it is part of *health* policy. The advantage of this is that mental health services will be considered and scrutinised by local managers and organisations such as the Commission for Health Improvement in much the same way as other parts of NHS. The drawback of this is that relevant agencies outside health which affect the quality of life of people with mental health problems (social services, housing, leisure, education, housing, voluntary sector providers, etc.) will not fall within its direct ambit, although a similar rationale is to be applied to social service departments. None the less, a large sector of agency involvement with clients (primary care and specialist mental health services) is within the NHS and so the policy of clinical governance is bound to have a high degree of salience in determining the *quality of service* received. Whether it impacts on clients' *quality of life* is a different question.

An unanswered question at present is whether clinical governance will control poor professional practice. One of the main architects of the policy was Liam Donaldson, the current Chief Medical Officer at the Department of Health. His interest prior to this role was in understanding and regulating poor *medical* practice ('poorly performing doctors'). This has a number of implications for mental health services. Psychiatrists are the least favoured professionals in the eyes of service-users (Rogers, Pilgrim and Lacey, 1993). The norms of acute psychiatric practice related to paternalism, poor communication skills and a narrow bio-medical approach evoke criticism in national and local user consultation exercises (Sainsbury Centre, 1998; Pilgrim and Hoser, 1999). Given the continuing pressures which keep psychiatrists in acute units in a paternalistic and controlling role it may be difficult for them to shift towards a more user-friendly norm. The problem is not always that they are 'poorly performing', which suggests that individual doctors are deviating from normal good practice; it may be that they are performing in a way which their professional training historically expected of them and current organisational pressures demand. Thus, if clinical governance is about raising quality as a user-defined outcome of services, then professional norms will need to change substantially in inpatient settings.

One of the building blocks of clinical governance is risk assessment and management. Potentially this is the one which might be easiest to implement efficiently because it can be governed by evidence-based protocols, which a multi-disciplinary group can 'sign up to'. The assessment and management of risky client behaviour is still more of an art than a science, especially in open settings. However, there is enough accumulated evidence about clinical, personality and actuarial variables to suggest that this aspect of clinical governance can be successful, given local managerial will. What is also open to protocol-driven improvements is the reduction of iatrogenic risk to clients. This is about seeing *professionals*, and not just clients, as risky (Pilgrim and Rogers, 1998). One example of improvement here is the control of poor drug prescribing. The latter includes: risky drug cocktails ('polypharmacy'); risky and unnecessary high dose levels ('megadosing'); and unresearched interventions. A good example in this last category is the tendency of clinicians to prescribe new drugs, such as the newer 'anti-psychotics', in combination with older drugs, even though the new drug is usually trialled for licence on its own (as a 'unitherapy'). Quality control over risky prescribing would place the profession of pharmacy centre-stage in this aspect of clinical governance.

A final implication of clinical governance which may be important in coming years is continuous professional development (CPD). As we noted in Chapter 5, a tension is emerging in health care systems about a managed approach to service quality based upon a multi-disciplinary commitment to practice guidelines (to promote cost-effectiveness) and one based on individual disciplines insisting on the control of their own professional standards and clinical practices. This tension comes out most strongly in relation to CPD. The first part of the tension will win the day if there is a collective commitment to multi-disciplinary training which is linked to collectively agreed and specified service aims and objectives. By contrast, if the traditional tribal or guild approach to training wins the day, then the desired aim of CPD contributing to raised service standards will be jeopardised.

The National Service Framework for Mental Health: *setting standards for services*

This document was issued by the Department of Health in October 1999. Its age focus was 18 to 65 years of age. Following an introduction to the rationale for service frameworks it spelled out five areas in which standards were to be set, namely, 'mental health promotion; primary care and access to services; effective services for people with severe mental illness; caring about carers; preventing suicide'. As two standards were announced each for primary care and for effective services, somewhat confusingly seven standards in total were set out for five areas.

The document made suggestions about the configuration of services. A strong emphasis was placed on the formation of dedicated mental health trusts in inner-city areas but other arrangements were to be permitted in more dispersed locations (i.e., community trusts or primary care trusts may carry mental health within a wider range of health services). Integration and inter-agency partnerships were to be emphasised and encouraged.

The process of production of the document entailed a variety of interests being alloyed. The main producers were a government-appointed external reference group (ERG), chaired by a social psychiatrist, Professor Graham Thornicroft, from the Institute of Psychiatry in London. He and another 42 people worked on the initial content of the report. They were drawn from the NHS, professional bodies, mental health research organisations and the voluntary sector. This inclusive 'stakeholder' involvement was then closed off by civil servants and government ministers. This second phase of production created an eight-month delay in the report's intended release date. The delay probably reflected tensions in the Department of Health about resources and the dilemma created by the ERG draft being more 'supportive' than 'safe' in its emphasis (reversing the message foregrounded in the sub-title of *Modernising Mental Health Services: Safe, Sound and Supportive*).

Having used the past tense to describe the production of the NSF, the present tense is now relevant because at the time of writing, and for the foreseeable future, the document represents the British government's formal prescription about what is expected of mental health services. The NSF generally reflects a set of compromises between the stakeholder interests on the ERG (from SANE and the National Schizophrenia Fellowship to MIND and Survivors Speak Out, and from the Royal College of Psychiatrists to the British Psychological Society). In addition, the long delay in the report's release suggests that government political interests were not readily or easily met by such a mixed stakeholder approach. Government ministers and their civil servant advisors were not prepared simply to accept and rubber stamp the will of the ERG. Instead, the first draft was subjected to extensive political scrutiny and control. The outcome is a strange admixture of academic writing, in which gradations of evidence are operationalised about points being made, to crude political rhetoric which seems to have been phrased by or for its political masters. Consequently, problems with the document include the following elements.

(1) *Mysterious authorship and confused discourse.* After the foreword by Frank Dobson, the then Secretary of State for Health, the document's authorship is immediately rendered mysterious. The language used in the body of the report is part academic appraisal and part political exhortation, and the reader does not know who produced which part. Because political interests in both the first and second phase of the production of the report shaped its eventual contents, any radical questioning of the nature of the mental health industry is expunged or omitted, as is any challenge to the contradictions of current government policy on mental health. For example, under the section on combating discrimination and exclusion, the following politically loaded statement is made: 'Most people are generally caring and sympathetic, but they are also concerned about the danger which they associate with a very small number of people with severe mental illness.' It then goes on to talk about reducing stigma via public education without reference to the prejudicial and exaggerated statements made about the link between dangerousness and mental health problems by government ministers. These statements explicitly pandered to and legitimised prejudice and discrimination. The contradiction (or hypocrisy) entailed in proposing social inclusion and combating discrimination against a background of prejudicial populist government strategies is there to see for the reader of the text. However, the contradiction is not reflected on or acknowledged in the NSF.

(2) *The status quo is legitimised.* With the exception of a recurring emphasis on a new primary care focus, there is no critical analysis of current service arrangements and why they are problematic. The focus on serious mental illness and vertical rather than horizontal relationships (about service access) suggests that reform of the current arrangements is all that is required. However, the depth of disaffection with current services reflected in the growth of anti-psychiatry and then the service-users' movement, and confirmed by user and carer research, does not come through in this document. Similarly, the social control role of the mental health industry is not addressed. Carers' interests are singled out but users' interests are not given the same salience.

(3) *The narrow and selective use of evidence.* This follows on from

the above two points. Broadly the evidence base for the report can be described as 'social-psychiatric' with a particular emphasis on the 'psychiatric'. Crude epidemiology is used, with no reflection on the extensive philosophical and social criticisms which have been made over decades about the conceptual problems of psychiatric theory and practice. Similarly, evidence about interventions is narrowly about current knowledge of technocentric treatments (pharmacological and psychological). The limits of this technocentric approach for a complex moral and political question like mental health are not discussed. For example, there is a wide knowledge-base about the sociology of mental health service access and community living. This type of mixed methodology research, which illuminates complex process issues, is barely touched upon, whereas the RCT approach to the treatment of illness is privileged. Again there is a clear failure to reflect upon the complexity of mental health in society.

Reform of the Mental Health Act 1983: Proposals for Consultation: *the CTO controversy*

This Green Paper (DH, 1999) was issued by the government in November 1999. It was based selectively upon the outcome of a scoping exercise about the need for new legislation commissioned by government in 1998. This expert scoping committee was chaired by an academic lawyer, Professor Genevra Richardson. The committee was not allowed to consider the abolition of mental health law but was asked to consider any issue related to reform of the 1983 Mental Health Act. Richardson reported to health ministers in July 1999 before both the Green Paper and the National Service Framework were issued. This policy vacuum was also constructed by another emerging joint policy from the Department of Health and the Home Office (about the management of dangerous people with severe personality disorder). Thus the scoping exercise was a serious academic review which rehearsed fundamental philosophical, as well as legal, aspects of mental health law. Despite this advantage of it being a government-sanctioned appraisal of the nature of legislation, it was cast from the outset as an advisory exercise. This was soon obvious when the Green Paper appeared.

The outcomes of the Richardson review and the Green Paper appeared simultaneously. The political significance of this was that the scoping exercise's fine details were instantly eclipsed and so not discussed at large by stakeholders in mental health debates before the

Green Paper itself. This would have been of little significance had the government endorsed the broad points considered in the Richardson review, but this was far from the case. All the options rehearsed by Richardson about the workings of any prospective legal arrangements were put in the context of a discussion about discrimination and patient autonomy. This wider, balancing, discussion was absent from the Green Paper. Differences between the Green Paper and the Richardson review highlight the fact that the government had a pretty fixed and pre-emptive agenda about legal reform which only had a narrow public safety focus. The items which demonstrate this point are set out below.

(1) *Non-discrimination.* The Richardson review recorded and acknowledged a point made by a number of parties consulted: namely, that mental health law is intrinsically discriminatory, as it singles out one group of people in society for consideration about their detention without trial. No other group is considered in this way. The review was forced to concede the government's stricture that abolition was not an option. It emphasised instead that where discrimination occurs it should be acknowledged and formally justified. No such discussion or need for justification appeared in the Green Paper.

(2) *Autonomy.* A second key point of principle highlighted by Richardson, but ignored in the Green Paper, was that of autonomy. If a break was to be made from medical (or any other form of) paternalism, then patient autonomy would need to be sensitively respected. In particular, the question of the capacity to refuse treatment was highlighted. It was argued by Richardson that the notion of capacity should be clarified and operationalised. By contrast, this question was ignored in the Green Paper in favour of prioritising considerations of risk in decision-making about patients. The wilful exclusion of a needed legal, moral and psychological discussion of the notion of capacity by the Green Paper created a further point about discrimination. The Green Paper emphasised the question of risk in a traditional paternalistic sense, as it refers once more to compulsory treatment orders being applied to those posing a risk to self or others. Risk to others entails danger to third parties and is thus subject to consideration of harm in the same way that, say, risk from a dangerous criminal might be judged. Thus risk to others is a legal consideration that is made about people other than those with mental health problems. However, risk to self is a completely different matter, as judgements and controlling actions are positively sanctioned and encouraged by mental health law which *only* applies to people with mental health problems. For example, alcohol

and tobacco use and mountaineering are not illegal. Even though these habits are known to be self-injurious, drinkers, smokers and mountaineers are not detained without trial. By contrast, people with mental health problems who may be at risk of harming themselves are open to such detention, even though suicide is not illegal in Britain and many nations noted above which are self-harming are tolerated or even socially rewarded. Thus the propensity for self-harm is dealt with by the State in a peculiar way, in the case of people with mental health problems. As a consequence mental health law, which allows detention without trial for self-harming behaviour, is intrinsically discriminatory.

(3) *Reciprocity*. This refers to the obligation of the State to provide adequate and effective specialist treatment, care and support for those whose liberty is removed. The principle of reciprocity was rehearsed in the Richardson review. The Green Paper did not reflect or reproduce this principle but, instead, it placed an emphasis on CTOs. The Green Paper ignored the advice from Richardson about the right to an assessment of a patient's mental health needs. Likewise, advice about a statutory right to early advocacy was rejected, as was the proposal that care teams should be obliged to aid patients in preparing advance statements. Thus all of the balancing advice of Richardson on reciprocity was ignored by government.

It soon became evident that many voluntary sector bodies were unhappy with the emphasis in the Green Paper on compulsion and its lesser emphasis upon the State's reciprocal duty of care. In the latter regard, the government carefully avoided any advice from Richardson which had resource implications about supporting and enabling patients. When the Green Paper was issued, protests about this uneven emphasis were made immediately by MIND, the National Schizophrenia Fellowship, the Manic Depressive Fellowship and the Mental Aftercare Association. This coalition handed in a petition of over 20 000 signatures to the Department of Health from users, relatives and professionals arguing for a policy of care for the majority rather than control for the few. The government received some support for its emphasis on CTOs from the Zito Trust and SANE. Both organisations had been associated for a number of years with an authoritarian or paternalistic stance about the need to control madness. (These are discussed later under the heading of micro processes.)

The contention about CTOs was not new. During the late 1980s, when a Conservative government toyed with introducing them, a sceptical and unsupportive reaction ensued from professionals. The Royal

College of Psychiatrists had come nearest to supporting them but even then ambivalently (because of splits in its ranks). Many professionals' objections were rehearsed again and registered in the Richardson review. Professionals were worried on several counts.

First, there was a concern that an explicitly controlling attitude in a community setting would lead to patients being alienated from services, thus leading to them avoiding or distrusting contact with professionals. Moreover, those at the radical-liberal end of the professions who wanted to uncouple the traditional social control function – which had been a part of mental health work since certification in the old asylums – from their caring and supportive role were seeking to reduce or eliminate, not enlarge, coercion in mental health work (see, e.g., Bracken and Thomas, 2000).

The second concern was about the practicalities of the orders. Whilst the government emphasised that the orders would be about removing people to a clinical setting to enforce treatment upon 'non-compliant' patients, a question remained about who precisely was to do the manhandling in a regular and lawful way. The Green Paper was vague on this point, noting only that such arrangements were to be recorded in a care plan.

A third objection was that held by the voluntary sector petitioners noted above. Compulsion was an easy political option when the State was being asked to provide resources for underfunded support services. A general suspicion held by many of those doubting the legitimacy of the compulsion emphasis in the Green Paper was that noted about *Modernising Mental Health Service*. Coercion is popular and vote catching, whereas a concern for civil liberties for a minority group (especially one with a dangerous image) can be a political liability. Moreover, the principle of reciprocity, if put into action, has fiscal implications. The Labour government of 1997 seeking re-election for a second term was producing a range of social policies which reflected these points. It wanted policy which minimised financial costs *but at the same time* was a populist strategy: it had to appeal to voters, even if it was to their common prejudices. The public safety emphasis in the Green Paper, combined with the omission of the principle of reciprocity (and its inevitable fiscal price) advocated by the Richardson review, confirmed that the government was indeed shaping its mental health policy within a broader strategy of electoral populism. There is no tax cost attached to ministerial appeals to fear and prejudice.

The rationale of CTOs is flawed on logical and empirical grounds. It assumes that compliance with treatment is actually effective. CTOs, without exception, refer to compliance with medication. CTOs offer only a specious sense of a technical fix for incorrigible madness when they rely on medication. Those who know anything about anti-psychotic medication are aware that it is ineffective in many cases and that many untreated cases have sane episodes. This is not like giving insulin to a diabetic, where a specific medicinal agent with a well understood physiological action can be titrated to give a specific and predictable beneficial effect. Diabetics who do not regularly receive their appropriate dose of insulin soon become ill and presently die. This type of unilinear prediction does not reliably apply to psychiatric patients accepting or receiving drug treatment. Psychiatric drugs are much cruder, with a wide variability across recipients in terms of both therapeutic and adverse effects.

A final empirical consideration comes from the USA where CTOs have been studied carefully. Swartz *et al.* (1999) found that community orders are not effective unless they are combined with a level of intense service contact. (In Chapter 9 we drew attention to this difficulty in the context of British norms of professional practice in community mental health work.)

Health Outcome Indicators: Severe Mental Illness *and the advice of academic social psychiatry*

This report, which appeared in 1999, was the outcome of a multidisciplinary group (including a user representative) looking at 'severe mental illness' (Charlwood *et al.*, 1999). It is part of a series organised and published by the National Centre for Health Outcome Developments, University of Oxford. (Other reports include indicators for a wide range of other diagnostic related groups including diabetes, breast cancer and stroke.)

The exact political status of the indicators are not clear at the time of writing. The foreword to the report immediately uses *A First Class Service* as its context of legitimacy, making an explicit claim that report 'concerns [its] third aspect-monitoring standards'. Although the groups were commissioned by the Department of Health and so retain its stamp of authority (literally on the report covers), their origins were under the previous Conservative administration. Thus the indicators have no clear government endorsement: for example, they are not alluded to in the NSF discussed above. None the less, the status of the academic stakeholder contributors gives the indicators an intrinsic legitimacy. To what degree they may or may not be used alongside the standards set by the NSF is not clear at present. As a further indication of the political ambiguity of the indicators, they draw upon previous work done by the Research Unit of the Royal College of Psychiatrists, in line with the previous government's *Health of the Nation* policy (Wing, Curtiss and Beevor, 1996). The report contains 20 indicators covering nine types of intervention, with the number of indicators given here in brackets (summarised from Charlwood *et al.*, 1999, 15):

- reduce or avoid the risk of severe mental illness (1)
- early detection of severe mental illness (1)
- maintain personal functioning and reduce the need for hospitalisation (4)
- restore functioning and reduce relapse rate, after hospital discharge (2)
- promote independent living and well-being (5)
- sustain collaboration between providers, users and carers (2)
- support carers and reduce their stress (1)
- ensure protection and good physical health of users (2)
- ensure protection of carers, service providers and the public (2)

The conceptual overlap with the standards set in the NSF can be seen in the above list. As with the NSF, the conceptual status of the DRG being considered is taken for granted and not problematised, although only the first two indicators rely explicitly on the notion of 'severe mental illness'. The rest of the indicators are about functions and processes, and are not diagnosis-led.

The point about the ambiguous legitimacy of policy guidance emerging under one government but commissioned by a previous, opposing, one was also pointed up in 1998 when the Fallon Inquiry into the functioning of Ashworth Special Hospital recommended its closure. Its advice was ignored pointedly by the Secretary of State for Health, Frank Dobson. The inquiry had been set up by the outgoing Conservative administration.

Micro Factors

In earlier chapters we drew attention to the micro processes of stakeholding (of professionals, users and 'carers'). The current and prospective implications of these for mental health policy in Britain will now be summarised under the following headings:

- guidelines and protocols versus uni-disciplinary interests
- morale, recruitment and retention

- professional adaptation to clinical governance
- the limits of user involvement and the users' movement
- the power of relatives

Guidelines and protocols versus uni-disciplinary interests

As we noted in the last section about meso factors, the practice guideline emphasis in health policy is now strong, mainly for reasons of improving cost-effectiveness and sometimes to ensure cost minimisation. The reason this is also a micro factor is that it relies on the local implementation of the principle by professionals. The latter vary in their enthusiasm for, or resistance against, a practice guideline policy shift. Inertia in organisational systems is well known, so custom and practice are often slow to change. Daily morale is often maintained in staff groups by an allegiance to the traditions of their peers and seniors. Thus even though guidelines and protocols may seem sensible on paper, staff co-operation with them is by no means guaranteed. It relies on a number of local factors, including effective intellectual leadership and active managerial support for change.

As well as the practice guideline movement stalling in the face of professional custom and practice, mental health is such a contested area that different professional groupings may compete for a dominant position about service ideology and task control.

Morale, recruitment and retention

In recent years staff recruitment and retention has been a problem in mental health services. This reflects a general problem, particularly in the NHS nursing workforce, and a specific problem about mental health services. With regard to the latter, there have been difficulties after large hospital run-down of dealing with the stress of the acute hospital regime with its high throughput and its emphasis on the management of risky behaviour. Suicide in acute units remains high. It is not uncommon for staff to find patients dead or dying by their own hand. They then face the ordeal of internal and external inquiries. The notion of a 'blame culture' in mental health services has thus become commonplace. Staff develop stress reactions, take sick leave and thus put pressure on those remaining at work. Some leave the service. This has taken place in a context in which there has been a continuous downward pressure from governments of both political hues to reduce suicide rates, making frontline staff feel personally responsible for a phenomenon (self-harm) which has multiple social causes.

Professional adaptation to clinical governance

At this stage we do not know how specific professions may adapt to clinical governance in particular local contexts. However, what we do know from the past about NHS performance is that clinical professionals do not mechanically and uniformly comply with policy dictated by central government. Externally imposed demands constitute both constraints or threats to professionals' interests *and* opportunities to extend those interests. As we noted above, a veiled agenda for clinical governance was the control of poorly-performing doctors. In psychiatry, especially inpatient work, 'poor performance' may be difficult to identify as the norms of practice have emerged in a context of the latent function of social control. In such circumstances, arbitrary decision-making and the discretionary powers of professionals have been common features of the pragmatics of daily clinical practice. This sets up ambiguous expectations about performance standards as staff are dealing with embodied irrationality, risky behaviour, situations in which 'something has to be done' and lawful state-delegated coercive powers. In these circumstances, the success of clinical governance and its contributory processes from clinical staff may be difficult to clarify unless three quite separate functions are audited in mental health services (Pilgrim, 1999): the amelioration of distress and the reduction of dysfunction; accommodation; and the control of risky behaviour. These three functions were housed together in the old asylums. Now they may be unreasonably demanded of acute inpatient units but reasonably expected of a comprehensive range of local mental health services.

The limits of user involvement and the users' movement

Whilst user-opposition to traditional psychiatric theory and practice has been common and globally widespread in the last 20 years, the British experience has had its peculiarities. The service-users' movement was late on the scene compared to other parts of Europe and North America (Rogers and Pilgrim, 1991). Moreover, it has been drawn into service matters around user-involvement in services splitting the energy and priorities of the movement. Government support for user-involvement was probably stronger under the Conservative administrations of the 1980s and early 1990s, when consumerism was an explicit ideological motif of public sector reform, including that of the NHS. By contrast, the Labour administration after 1997 placed its emphasis upon other priorities such as improving equitable access, controlling service quality via clinical governance, 'caring for carers' and public safety

(DH, 1998, 1999c). The last on the list has been given the highest profile in ministerial statements about mental health policy. This has had a demoralising effect upon the users' movement.

The tendency of the new Labour administration to reinforce public prejudice about psychiatric patients has led to anger from some in the movement. For example, user-representatives invited on to the Internal Reference Group on mental health set up by the Government resigned very publicly at the 1998 annual MIND conference. They and their supporters heckled John Hutton, the minister newly-responsible for mental health, when he was speaking at the conference and it soon became evident that Labour's attitude towards users was decidedly ambivalent. Although the NSF, published in 1999, argued that 'specific arrangements should be in place to ensure service-user and carer involvement', the user allusion fades from view later in the document with the exception of one brief mention of a 'beacon service' of user-support (DH, 1999c, 60). Standard six in the NSF is about caring for carers; users are not mentioned in the section elaborating the point. The governmental restrictions imposed upon service-users after 1997 joined a list of other constraints and opportunities extant in late modernity in the developed world (Pilgrim and Waldron, 1998).

The power of relatives

Lobbies dominated by relatives have had a clear influence upon governments, past and present. A good example of this is the work of SANE, whose leader Marjorie Wallace, an ex-*Times* journalist, has been skilful in impressing upon ministers in the Department of Health the dangers of an overly-liberal attitude towards patients' rights. The SANE campaign over the past ten years has emphasised how dangerous patients can be and how much they as sick individuals require greater enforced hospitalisation and treatment. The theme of dangerousness has also been salient in the work of the Zito Trust, headed by Jayne Zito; the man who murdered her husband was sent to Rampton high security hospital following his trial. By contrast in recent years the work of another relatives-dominated group, the National Schizophrenia Fellowship, has shifted away from one opposing hospital run-down and closure in the mid-1980s to one which places more of an emphasis upon a well-resourced range of services. Whilst much overlap exists between the demands of relatives' groups and users' groups, as we noted in Chapter 6, their interests at times can be discrepant.

As was noted above, the power of relatives is represented explicitly and formally in Standard six of the NSF ('caring for carers'). This will have given a fillip to relatives' groups in their local campaigns to change services. Apart from campaigning, relatives' groups have also become substantial service-providers. For example, the National Schizophrenia Fellowship and a derivative group in the North of England (Making Space) are now established providers of aftercare in the voluntary sector, running hostels and sheltered housing and employing support and development workers.

Conclusion

This final chapter provides the reader with a contemporary sense of British mental health policy. It offers a different picture from that written for the first edition of this book, suggesting that policy descriptions are necessarily temporary and provisional. However, the macro factors we introduced at the outset also suggest a sort of continuity. There is a pattern that connects over time and across different societies. This, more enduring, picture is characterised by Rosen's point (1968) about aimless wandering and violence. The point suggests a recurring concern about madness in any society, even if the way it is constructed by religious and secular experts varies to some degree over time and place. Whether in ancient regimes or modern, individualist or collectivist, madness and its associated lack of intelligibility, irrationality and subversiveness offends the daily social contract. This point is elaborated here by Jonathan Miller:

> It appears in the family first and then of course it appears in public places. There is a vast, very complicated, unwritten constitution of conduct which allows us to move with confidence through public spaces, and we can instantly and by a very subtle process recognise someone who is breaking that constitution. They're talking to themselves; they're not moving at the same rate; they're moving at different angles; they're not avoiding other people with the skill that pedestrians do in the street. The speed with which normal users of public places can recognise someone else as not being a normal user of it is where madness appears. (Miller, 1991, 31)

Madness is not the only form of deviance. For example, intoxication, sexual deviation, dimness, violent and non-violent criminality, genius and creativity have domains which can be described separately and when they overlap. However, the challenge to the social order madness emerges within provokes a peculiar mixture of pity, exasperation and fear in its onlookers. This reactive state invites them to tolerate or control its expression. The range of possibilities this sets up for politicians and their lay supporters about 'mental health policy' inevitably creates tensions about tolerance (expressed by civil libertarians) and control (expressed by paternalists).

When we turn away from madness to consider the wider modern connotation of 'mental health problems' then Rosen's point is less pertinent, or at least it only partially defines the concept of 'mental health policy'. Newer considerations have to be added to the traditional frustrations and fears incorrigible madness provokes. As was noted at the start of this chapter, it is common in Britain and other developed countries also to include questions of 'mental health promotion'. That is, an important aspect of modernity is the expectation that citizens will enjoy a positive sense of well-being, not merely an absence of illness. Also, during the twentieth century, professional jurisdiction over 'minor' mental health problems, generally called the 'neuroses', has increasingly occupied the interest of general practitioners, counsellors and psychological therapists of different theoretical persuasions. This general category covers a group of people who cause little offence to others but who are, in various ways, miserable.

A final category that connects the nineteenth-century emphasis on problems to others (lunacy) and the twentieth-century emphasis on problems to the self (neurosis) is that of 'personality disorder'. This contentious rag-bag category includes what was first called 'moral insanity' (by Morel in 1864) and is now called 'anti-social personality disorder' under DSM-IV and 'psychopathic disorder' under ICD10. It also includes a range of other sub-types which in a variety of ways allude to inter-personal dysfunction. This range subsumes features of offence to others and distress in those receiving the diagnosis.

Thus the term 'mental health policy' (in most developed societies including Britain) at the turn of the twenty-first century refers to legal arrangements, policy directives and service investments in relation to the aggregate picture just described, which have accumulated over the past hundred years. It is partly about the control of mad behaviour, partly about promoting well-being, partly about ameliorating distress and partly about responding to dysfunction. Given such a wide remit, it is hardly surprising that the notion of mental health policy is now highly ambiguous. A century ago such an ambiguity did not exist: there was a basically a *lunacy policy*, with segregation (the asylum system) being the single total organisational solution. As we noted in Chapter 3, the First World War changed this picture and, nearly a century later, mental health policy reflects more and more contestation, both in our definitions and theories of psychological normality and abnormality and in our political responses to them.

Bibliography

Abel, B. (1988) *The British Legal Profession* (Oxford: Basil Blackwell).

Abel-Smith, B. (1960) *A History of the Nursing Profession* (London: Heinemann).

Abramson, M. (1972) 'The criminalisation of mentally disordered behaviour: possible side-effects of a new mental health law', *Hospital and Community Psychiatry*, 23(3), pp. 101–5.

Acheson, D. (1998) *Independent Inquiry into Inequalities in Health* (London: HMSO).

Akilu, F. (1991) 'Women's experience of homelessness', *Newsletter of the Psychology of Women's Section of the British Psychological Society*, 8, pp. 1–12.

Alford, R. (1975) *Health Care Politics* (Chicago: University of Chicago Press).

Allderidge, P. (1979) 'Hospitals, madhouses and asylums: cycles in the care of the insane', *British Journal of Psychiatry*, 34, pp. 321–34.

Allness, D. J. and Knoedler, W. H. (1999) *The PACT Model of Community-Based Treatment for Persons with Severe and Persistent Mental Illnesses* (Arlington, Virginia: National Association of Mental Illness).

Allsop, J. (1984) *Health Policy and the National Health Service* (London: Longman).

Andreason, N. (1989) 'The scale for the assessment of negative symptoms (SANS): conceptual and theoretical foundations', *British Journal of Psychiatry*, Supplement 7, 155, pp. 49–52.

Appleby, L., Cooper, J., Amos, T. and Faragher, M. (1999a) Psychological autopsy study of suicides by people aged under 35, British Journal of Psychiatry 175, pp, 168–74.

Appleby, L., Shaw, J., Amos, T., McDonnell, R., Harris, C., McCann, K., Kieran, K., Davies, S., Bickly, H. and Parsons, R. (1999b) 'Suicide within 12 months of contact with mental health services: national clincial survey', *British Medical Journal*, 318, pp. 1235–9.

Armstrong, D. (1979) 'The emancipation of biographical medicine', *Social Science and Medicine*, 13, pp. 1–8.

Armstrong, D. (1980) 'Madness and coping', *Sociology of Health and Illness*, 2(3), pp. 393–413.

Ashton, J. (1990) 'Creating healthy cities', in C. Martin and D. McQueen (eds), *Readings for a New Public Health* (Edinburgh: Edinburgh University Press).

Ashton, J. and Seymour, H. (1988) *The New Public Health* (Milton Keynes: Open University Press).

Atkinson, P. (1983) 'The reproduction of the professional community', in R. Dingwall and P. Lewis (eds), *The Sociology of the Professions* (London: Macmillan).

Audit Commission (1986) *Making a Reality of Community Care* (London: Audit Commission).

Audit Commission (1994) *Finding a Place* (London: Audit Commission).

Balint, M. (1957) *The Doctor, His Patient and the Illness* (London: Tavistock).

Barham, P. and Hayward, R. (1991) *From the Mental Patient to the Person* (London: Routledge).

Barker, I. and Peck, E. (eds) (1987) *Power in Strange Places* (London: Good Practices in Mental Health).

Barnes, M. (1999) 'Users as citizens: collective action and the local governance of welfare', *Social Policy and Administration*, 33(1), pp. 73–90.

Barnes, M., Bowl, R. and Fisher, M. (1990) *Sectioned: Social Services and the 1983 Mental Health Act* (London: Routledge).

Barnes, M. and Maple, N. (1992) *Women and Mental Health: Challenging the Stereotypes* (Birmingham: Venture Press).

Barron, C. (1988) *Asylum to Anarchy* (London: FAB).

Barton, W. R. (1959) *Institutional Neurosis* (Bristol: Wright & Sons).

Baruch, G. and Treacher, A. (1978) *Psychiatry Observed* (London: Routledge & Kegan Paul).

Basaglia, F. (1981) 'Breaking the circuit of control', in D. Ingleby (ed.), *Critical Psychiatry* (Harmondsworth: Penguin).

Bassuk, E., Rubin, L. and Lauriat, A. (1984) 'Is homelessness a mental health problem?', *American Journal of Psychiatry*, 141, pp. 1546–50.

Baughan, R. (1993) *Suicide: A Summary of Different Approaches and Perspectives* (Banstead: COHSE).

Bean, P. (1979) 'Psychiatrists' assessments of mental illness: a comparison of Thomas Scheff's approach to labelling theory', *British Journal of Psychiatry*, 135, pp. 122–8.

Bean, P. (1980) *Compulsory Admissions to Mental Hospital* (Chichester: Wiley).

Bean, P. (1985) 'Social control and social theory in secure accommodation', in L. Gostin (ed.), *Secure Provision* (London: Tavistock).

Bean, P. (1986) *Mental Disorder and Legal Control* (Cambridge: Cambridge University Press).

Bean, P., Bingley, W., Bynoe, L., Faulkner, A., Rassaby, E. and Rogers, A. (1991) *Out of Harm's Way* (London: MIND).

Bean, P. and Mounser, P. (1993) *Discharged from Mental Hospitals* (London: Macmillan).

Beardshaw, V. and Morgan, E. (1990) *Community Care Works* (London: MIND)

Beattie, A. (1991) 'Knowledge and control in health promotion: a test case for social policy and social theory', in J. Gabe, M. Calnan and M. Bury (eds), *The Sociology of the Health Service* (London: Routledge).

Beazley, M. (1994) 'Measuring service quality', in N. Malin (ed.), *Implementing Community Care* (Buckingham: Open University Press).

Bebbington, P. E., Hurry, J. and Tennant, C. (1981) 'Psychiatric disorders in selected immigrant groups in Camberwell', *Social Psychiatry*, 16, pp. 43–51.

Beliappa, J. (1991) *Illness or Distress? Alternative Models of Mental Health* (London: Confederation of Indian Organisations).

Bentall, R., Day, J., Rogers, A., Healy, D. and Stevenson, R. (1996) 'Side effects of neuroleptic medication: assessment and impact on outcome of psychotic disorders', in S. Moscarelli, A. Rupp and N. Sartorius (eds), *The Economics of Schizophrenia* (London: Wiley).

Bentall, R., Jackson, H. and Pilgrim, D. (1998) 'Abandoning the concept of schizophrenia: some implications of validity arguments for psychological research into psychosis', *British Journal of Clinical Psychology*, 27, pp. 303–24.

Beresford, P. and Croft, S. (1986) *Whose Welfare? Private Care or Public Service* (London: Lewis Cohen Urban Studies).

Bergin, A. E. and Garfield, S. L. (1994) *Handbook of Psychotherapy and Behavior Change* (New York: Wiley).

Berridge, V., Webster, C. and Walt, G. (1993) 'Mobilisation for total welfare 1948–1974', in C. Webster (ed.), *Caring for Health: History and Diversity* (Buckingham: Open University Press).

Beutler, L., Machado, P. and Neufeldt, S. (1994) 'Therapist variables', in A. E. Bergin and S. L. Garfield (eds), *Handbook of Psychotherapy and Behavior Change* (New York: Wiley).

Bindman, J., Beck, A., Glover, G., Thornicroft, G., Knapp, M., Leese, M. and Szmukler, G. (1999) 'Evaluating mental health policy in England: Care Programme Approach and Supervision Registers', *British Journal of Psychiatry*, 35, pp. 327–30.

Bion, W. (1958) *Experiences in Groups* (London: Tavistock).

Blaxter, M. (1990) *Health and Lifestyles* (London: Routledge).

Bleuler, E. (1911) *Dementia Praecox or the Groups of Schizophrenias* (English edn, 1955) (New York: International Universities Press).

Bloch, S. and Reddaway, P. (1977) *Psychiatric Terror: How Soviet Psychiatry is Used to Suppress Dissent* (New York: Basic Books).

Blom-Cooper, L. and Murphy, E. (1991) 'Mental health services and resources', *Psychiatric Bulletin*, 15, pp. 65–8.

Bluglass, R. (1985) 'The development of regional secure units', in L. Gostin (ed.), *Secure Provision* (London: Tavistock).

Bolton, P. (1984) 'Management of compulsorily admitted patients to a high security unit', *International Journal of Social Psychiatry*, 30, pp. 77–84.

Bower, P. and Sibbald, B. (1999) 'On-site mental health workers in primary care: effects on professional practice. Protocol for a Cochrane Review', in *The Cochrane Library*, Issue 3 (Oxford: Update Software).

Bowlby, J. (1969) *Attachment* (London: Hogarth Press).

Bracken, P., and Thomas, P., (1998) 'A new debate in mental health', *Open Mind* 89, February, p. 17.

Bradley, P. and Hirsch, S. (eds) (1986) *The Psychopharmacology and Treatment of Schizophrenia* (Oxford: Oxford University Press).

Bradshaw, J. (1994) 'The conceptualisation and measurement of need: a social policy perspective', in J. Popay and G. Williams (eds), *Researching the People's Health* (London: Routledge).

Breggin, P. (1993) *Toxic Psychiatry* (London: Fontana).

British Medical Association (1938) *A General Medical Service for the Nation* (London: BMA).

Brown, G. W. (1959) 'Experiences of discharged chronic schizophrenic patients in various types of living group', *Millbank Memorial Fund Quarterly*, 37, p. 105.

Brown, G. W. (1973) 'The mental hospital as an institution', *Social Science and Medicine*, 7, pp. 407–21.

Brown, G. W., Birley, J. and Wing, J. K. (1972) 'Influence of family life on the course of schizophrenic disorders: a replication', *British Journal of Psychiatry*, 121, pp. 241–58.

Brown, G. W., Bone, M., Dalison, B. and Wing, J. K. (1966) *Schizophrenia and Social Care: A Comparative Follow-Up of 339 Schizophrenic Patients*, Maudsley Monograph no. 17 (London: Oxford University Press).

Brown, G. W. and Harris, T. O. (1978) *The Social Origins of Depression* (London: Tavistock).

Brown, G. W., Harris, T. O. and Bifulco, A. (1986) 'Long term effects of early loss of parent', in M. Rutter, C. Izard, and P. Read (eds), *Depression In Childhood: Developmental Perspectives* (New York: Guildford Press).

Brown, G. W. and Wing, J. K. (1962) 'A comparative clinical and social survey of three mental hospitals', *The Sociological Review Monograph*, 5, pp. 145–71.

Brown, P. and Funk, S. C. (1986) 'Tardive dyskinesia: barriers to the professional recognition of iatrogenic disease', *Journal of Health and Social Behaviour*, 27, pp. 116–32.

Browne, A. and Finklehor, D. (1986) 'Impact of child sexual abuse: a review of the research', *Psychological Bulletin*, 99, pp. 66–77.

Browne, D. (1990) *Black People, Mental Health and the Courts* (London: NACRO).

Bruce, M. L., Takeuchi, D. T. and Keaf, P. L. (1991) 'Poverty and psychiatric status', *Archives of General Psychiatry*, 48, pp. 470–4.

Brugha, T. and Lindsay, F. (1996) 'Quality of mental health service care: The forgotten pathway from process to outcome', *Social Psychiatry and Psychiatric Epidemiology*, 31, pp. 89–98.

Bryers, J. B., Nelson, B. A., Miller J. B. and Krol, P.A. (1987) 'Childhood sexual and physical abuse as factors in adult psychiatric illness', *American Journal of Psychiatry*, 144, pp. 1426–31.

Buetow, S. A. and Roland, M. (1999) 'Clinical governance: bridging the gap betweeen managerial and clinical approaches to quality of care', *Quality in Health Care*, 8, pp. 184–90.

Burns, T., Creed, F., Fahy, T., Thompson, S., Tyrer, P. and White, I. (1999) 'Intensive versus standard case management for severe psychotic illness. A randomised trial', *Lancet*, 353, pp. 2185–9.

Burrows, W. (1969) 'Community psychiatry – another bandwagon?', *Journal of the Canadian Psychiatric Association*, 14, pp. 105–14.

Burstow, B. and Weitz, D. (eds) (1988) *Shrink Resistant: The Struggle Against Psychiatry in Canada* (Vancouver: New Star Books).

Bury, M. and Gabe, J. (1990) 'Hooked? Media responses to tranquillizer dependence', in P. Abbott and G. Payne (eds), *New Directions in the Sociology of Health* (London: Falmer Press).

Busfield, J. (1982) 'Gender and mental illness', *International Journal of Mental Health*, 11(1–2), pp. 46–66.

Busfield, J. (1986) *Managing Madness* (London: Hutchinson).

Busfield, J. (1988) 'Mental illness as a social product or social construct: a contradiction in feminists' arguments?', *Sociology of Health and Illness*, 10, pp. 521–42.

Byalin, K. (1991) 'The quality assurance dilemma in psychiatry: a sociological perspective', *Community Mental Health Journal*, 28, pp. 453–9.

Cahill, M. (1994) *The New Social Policy* (Oxford: Basil Blackwell).

Callanan, M., Dunne, T., Morris, D. and Stern, R. (1997) *Primary Care, Serious*

Mental Illness and the Local Community: Developing a Commissioning Framework (Tunbridge, Kent: Salomons Centre).

Calnan, M. and Gabe, J. (1991) 'Recent developments in general practice: a sociological analysis', in J. Gabe *et al.*, *The Sociology of the Health Service* (London: Routledge).

Campbell, T. and Heginbotham, C. (1991) *Mental Illness, Prejudice Discrimination and the Law* (Aldershot: Dartmouth).

Carmen, E. H., Ricker, P.P. and Mills, T. (1984) 'Victims of violence and psychiatric illness', *American Journal of Psychiatry*, 141, pp. 378–83.

Carpenter, I. and Brockington, I. (1980) 'A study of mental illness in Asians, West Indians and Africans living in Manchester', *British Journal of Psychiatry*, 137, pp. 201–5.

Carpenter, M. (1980) 'Asylum nursing before 1914: a chapter in the history of labour', in C. Davies (ed.), *Rewriting Nursing History* (London: Croom Helm).

Carpenter, M. (1994a) 'Community Care: the "other" health reform', *Medical Sociology News*, 19(2), pp. 30–3.

Carpenter, M. (1994b) *Normality is Hard Work* (London: Lawrence & Wishart).

Castel, R., Castel, R. and Lovell, A. (1979) *The Psychiatric Society* (New York: Columbia Free Press).

Catalan, J., Gath, D. H. and Bond, A. (1988) 'General practice patients on long term psychotropic drugs: a controlled investigation', *British Journal of Psychiatry*, 152, pp. 263–8.

Chamberlin, J. (1988) *On Our Own* (London: MIND).

Charlwood, B. *et al.* (1999) *Health Outcome Indicators: Severe Mental Illness* (Oxford: National Centre for Health Outcome Developments).

Chapple, A., Rogers, A., McDonald, W. and Sergison, M. (2000) Patients' perceptions of changing professional boundaries and the future of 'nurse-led' services, *Primary Care Research and Development*, 1: 49–57.

Chen, E., Harrison, G. and Standen, P. (1991) 'Management of first episode psychotic illness in Afro-Caribbean patients', *British Journal of Psychiatry*, 158, pp. 517–22.

Chesler, P. (1972) *Women and Madness* (New York: Doubleday).

Ciompi, L. (1984) 'Is there really a schizophrenia? The long term course of psychotic phenomena', *British Journal of Psychiatry*, 145, pp. 636–40.

Clare, A. (1976) *Psychiatry in Dissent* (London: Tavistock).

Clausen, J. A. and Kohn, M. L. (1959) 'Relation of schizophrenia to the social structure of a small city', in B. Pasamanick (ed.), *Epidemiology of Mental Disorders* (Washington, DC: American Association for the Advancement of Science).

Clegg, S. R. (1990) *Modern Organisations* (London: Sage).

Clements, J. (1994) 'Comment', *OpenMind*, 3, p. 70.

Cobb, A. and Wallcraft, J. (1989) 'Women's needs', in A. Brackx and C. Grimshaw (eds), *Mental Health Care in Crisis* (London: Pluto Press).

Cochrane, D. (1988) '"Humane, economical, and medically wise": the LCC as administrators of Victorian lunacy policy', in W. Bynan, R. Porter and M. Shepherd (eds), *The Anatomy of Madness: Essays in the History of Psychiatry* (London: Routledge).

Cochrane, R. (1977) 'Mental illness in immigrants to England and Wales:

an analysis of mental hospital admissions 1971', *Social Psychiatry*, 12, pp. 2–35.

Cochrane, R. and Bal, S. (1989) 'Mental hospital admission rates of immigrants to England: a comparison of 1971 and 1981', *Social Psychiatry*, 24, pp. 2–11.

Cohen, D., (1997) 'A critique of the use of neuroleptic drugs in psychiatry', in S. Fisher and R. P. Greenberg (eds), *From Placebo to Panacea* (New York: Wiley).

Community Psychiatric Nurses' Association (1988) *The Patient's Case* (London: CPNA).

Cooper, B., Harwin, B. and Depla, C. (1975) 'Mental health care in the community: an evaluative study', *Psychological Medicine*, 5, pp. 372–80.

Cooper, D. (1968) *Psychiatry and Anti-Psychiatry* (London: Tavistock).

Cooperstock, R. (1978) 'Sex differences in psychotropic drug use', *Social Science and Medicine*, 12, pp. 179–86.

Cope, R. (1989) 'The compulsory detention of Afro-Caribbeans under the Mental Health Act', *New Community*, 15(3), pp. 343–56.

Copeland, J., Dewey, M., Wodd, N., Searle, R., Davidson, I. and McWilliam, C. (1987) 'Range of mental illness among the elderly in the community', *British Journal of Psychiatry*, 150, pp. 815–23.

Coulter, J. (1973) *Approaches to Insanity* (New York: Wiley).

Crawford, D. (1989) 'The future of clinical psychology: whither or wither?', *Clinical Psychology Forum*, 20, pp. 29–31.

Creed, F. and Marks, B. (1989) 'Liaison psychiatry in general practice', *Journal of Royal College of General Practitioners*, 39, pp. 514–17.

Crepaz-Keay, D. (1994) '"I wish to register a complaint . . ."', *OpenMind*, 71, pp. 4–5.

Crompton, R. (1987) 'Gender, status and professionalism', *Sociology*, 21(3), pp. 413–28.

Crystel, S., Ladner, S. and Towber, R. (1986) 'Multiple impairment patterns in the mentally ill homeless', *International Journal of Mental Health*, 14, pp. 61–73.

Curran, W. (1979) 'Comparative analysis of mental health legislation in forty-three countries: a discussion of historical trends', *International Journal of Law and Psychiatry*, 1(1), pp. 79–92.

Curtis, J. L., Millman, E. J. and Struening, E. (1992) 'Effect of case management on re-hospitalisation and utilisation of ambulatory care services', *Hospital and Community Psychiatry*, 43, pp. 895–9.

Dabbs, A. (1972) 'The changing role of clinical psychologists in the National Health Service', *Bulletin of the British Psychological Society*, 26, pp. 123–7.

Dalley, G. (1988) *Ideologies of Caring* (London: Macmillan).

Davidge, M., Elias, S., Jayes, B., Wood, K. and Yates, J. (1993) *Survey of English Mental Illness Hospitals* (University of Birmingham: Inter-Authority Comparisons and Consultancy Health Services Management Centre).

Davidhazar. D. and Wehlage, D. (1984) 'Can the client with chronic schizophrenia consent to nursing research?', *Journal of Advanced Nursing*, 9, pp. 381–90.

Davis, A., Llewellyn, S. P. and Parry, G. (1985) 'Women and mental health: a guide for the Approved Social Worker', in E. Brook and A. Davis (eds), *Women, the Family and Social Work* (London: Tavistock).

Dawson Report (1920) *Report of the Consultative Council on Medical and Allied Services* (London: Ministry of Health).

De Boer, F. (1991) 'Sex differences in the construction of mental health care problems', paper presented at the British Sociological Association Medical Sociology Conference, York.

De Swaan A. (1990) *The Management of Normality* (London: Routledge).

Dean, G. and Gadd, D. M. (1990) 'Home treatment for acute psychiatric illness', *British Medical Journal*, 301, pp. 1021–3.

Dean, G., Walsh, D., Downing, H. and Shelly, P. (1981) 'First admission of native-born and immigrants to psychiatric hospitals in South-East England 1976', *British Journal of Psychiatry*, 139, pp. 506–12.

Dennis, J., Draper, P., Holland. S., Snipster, P., Speller, V. and Sunter, J. (1982) 'Health promotion in the reorganised NHS', *The Health Services Journal*, 26 November.

DH (1989) *Health and Personal Social Service Statistics* (London: HMSO).

DH (1992a) *Health and Personal Social Service Statistics* (London: HMSO).

DH (1992b) *The Health of the Nation* (London: HMSO).

DH (1994a) *Health and Personal Social Services Statistics for England*. NHS Workforce in England Edition (London: HMSO).

DH (1994b) *Mental Health Task Force, Local Systems of Support: A Framework for Purchasing for People with Severe Mental Health Problems* (London: HMSO).

DH (1994c) *NHS Workforce in England* (London: HMSO).

DH (1994d) Press Release 94/526 *Two New Publications on Mental Health Needs of People from Ethnic Minority Communities* (London: DH).

DH (1994e) *Working in Partnership: A Collaborative Approach to Care* (London: HMSO).

DH (1995) *Building Bridges* (London: HMSO).

DH (1997a) *The New NHS: Modern and Dependable* (London: HMSO).

DH (1998) *Modernising Mental Health Services: Safe, Sound and Supportive* (London: HMSO).

DH (1998) *Our Healthier Nation* (London: HMSO).

DH (1999a) 'Inpatients formally detained in hospitals under the Mental Health Act 1983 and other legislation, England: 1988–89 to 1998–99', *Statistical Bulletin* (London: DH).

DH (1999b) *Effective Care Co-Ordination in Mental Health Services: Modernising the Care Programme Approach* (London: HMSO).

DH (1999c) *National Service Framework for Mental Health* (London: HMSO).

DH (1999d) *Reform of the Mental Health Act 1983* (London: DH).

DH (1999e) *A First Class Service* (London: DH).

DHSS (1971) *Enquiry into the Practice and Effects of Scientology* (The Foster Report) (London: HMSO).

DHSS (1975) *Better Services for the Mentally Ill* (London: HMSO).

DHSS (1977) *The Role of Psychologists in the Health Service* (The Trethowan Report) (London: HMSO).

DHSS (1980) *Inequalities in Health: Report of a Working Group* (London: HMSO).

DHSS (1980a) *Organisation and Management Problems of Mental Illness Hospitals* (The Nodder Report) (London: HMSO).

DHSS (1980b) *Report of the Review of Rampton Hospital* (London: HMSO).

DHSS (1987) *Mental Illness and Mental Handicap Hospitals and Units in England: Legal Statistics 1982–85*, DHSS Statistical Bulletin 2/87 (London: HMSO).

DHSS (1988) *Report of the Committee of Inquiry into the Care and After-care of Miss Sharon Campbell*, Cmnd440 (London: HMSO).

Dick, P. H., Sweeney, M. L. and Crombie, I. K. (1991) 'Controlled comparison of day patient and outpatient treatment for persistent anxiety and depression', *British Journal of Psychiatry*, 158, pp. 24–7.

Dietzen, L. L. and Bond, G. R. (1993) 'Relationship between case manager contact and outcome for frequently hospitalised psychiatric clients', *Hospital and Community Psychiatry*, 44, pp. 839–43.

Dobson, F. (1998) 'Frank Dobson outlines third way for mental health', DH Press Release (London: DH).

Dobson, K. S. and Craig, K. D. (eds) *Empirically Supported Therapies* (London: Sage).

Dohrenwend, B. and Dohrenwend, S. (eds) (1974) *Stressful Life Events: Their Nature and Effects* (New York: John Wiley).

Donnelly, M. (1983) *Managing the Mind* (London: Tavistock).

Donzelot, J. (1980) *The Policing of Families* (London: Hutchinson).

Doyal, L. and Gough, I. (1991) *A Theory of Human Need* (London: Macmillan).

Dunham, H. W. (1964) 'Social class and schizophrenia', *American Journal of Orthopsychiatry*, 34, pp. 634–46.

Dunham, H. W. (1967) 'Community psychiatry the newest therapeutic bandwagon', *Current Issues in Psychiatry*, 5, pp. 612–13 (New York: Science House).

DYG Corporation (1990) *Public Attitudes toward People with Chronic Mental Illness* (Elmsford, NY: DYG Corporation).

Earl, L. and Kincey, J. (1982) 'Clinical psychology in general practice: a controlled trial evaluation', *Journal of the Royal College of General Practice*, 32, pp. 32–7.

Easton, D. (1953) *The Political System* (New York: Knopf).

Edwards, M. and Fasal, J. (1992) 'Keeping an intimate relationship professional', *OpenMind*, 57, pp. 10–11.

Ennis, B. and Emery, R. (1978) *The Rights of Mental Patients – An American Civil Liberties Union Handbook* (New York: Avon).

Eppel, A. B., Fuyarchuk, C., Pheips, D. and Tersigni-Phelen, A. (1991) 'A comprehensive and practical quality assurance program for community mental health services', *Canadian Journal of Psychiatry*, 36, pp. 102–6.

Estroff, S. and Zimmer, C. (1994) 'Social networks, social support, and violence among persons with severe, persistent mental illness', in J. Monahan and H. Steadman (eds), *Violence and Mental Disorder: Developments in Risk Assessment* (Chicago: University of Chicago Press).

Etzioni, A. (1995) *The Spirit of Community* (London: Fontana).

Falloon, I. and Fadden, G. (1993) *Integrated Mental Health Care* (Cambridge: Cambridge University Press).

Farmer, A. and Griffiths, H. (1992) 'Labelling and illness in primary care: comparing factors influencing general practitioners' and psychiatrists' decisions regarding patient referral to mental illness services', *Psychological Medicine*, 22, pp. 717–23.

Farris, R. E. L. (1994) 'Ecological factors in human behaviour', in R. E. L. Farris and H. W. Dunham, *Mental Disorders in Urban Areas: An Ecological Study of Schizophrenia* (Chicago: Chicago University Press).

Faulkner, A. (1992) 'Planned Provision Blues', *Community Care*, 22 (Oct.), pp. 20–1.

Fennell, P. (1991) 'Diversion of mentally disordered offenders from custody', *Criminal Law Review*, 1, pp. 333 10.

Fenton, S. and Sadiq, A. (1991) *Asian Women and Depression* (London: Commission for Racial Equality).

Ferguson, B. and Varnam, M. (1994) 'The relationship between primary care and psychiatry: an opportunity for change', *British Journal of General Practice*, 44, pp. 527–30.

Fernando, S. (1988) *Race and Culture in Psychiatry* (London: Routledge).

Fernando, S. (1992) 'Psychiatry', *OpenMind*, 58, pp. 8–9.

Field Institute (1984) *In Pursuit of Wellness: A Survey of California Adults* (Sacramento: California Department of Mental Health).

Finch, J. and Groves, D. (1980) 'Community care and the family: a case for equal opportunities', *Journal of Social Policy*, 9, p. 4.

Finn, S. E., Bailey, M., Schultz, R. T. and Faber, R. (1990) 'Subjective utility ratings of neuroleptics in treating schizophrenia', *Psychological Medicine*, 20, pp. 843–8.

Fisher, S. R. and Greenberg, P. (eds) (1997) *From Placebo to Panacea: Putting Psychiatric Drugs to the Test* (New York: Wiley).

Forsythe, B. (1990) 'Mental and social diagnosis and the English Prison Commission 1914–1939', *Social Policy and Administration*, 24(3), pp. 237–53.

Foucault, M. (1961) *Folie et deraison: histoire de la folie a l'age classique* (Paris: Plon).

Foucault, M. (1964) *Madness and Civilisation* (New York: Random House).

Foucault, M. (1988) 'Technologies of the self', in L. Martin (ed.), *The Technologies of the Self* (London: Tavistock).

Francis, E. (1989) 'Black people, dangerousness and psychiatric compulsion', in A. Brackx and C. Grimshaw (eds), *Mental Health Care in Crisis* (London: Pluto).

Francis, E., Pilgrim, D., Rogers, A. and Sashidaran, S. (1989) 'Race and "schizophrenia": a reply to Ineichen', *New Community*, 3, pp. 161–3.

Franklin, J. L., Solovitz, B. and Mason, M. (1981) 'An evaluation of case management', *American Journal of Public Health*, 4, pp. 674–8.

Frederick, J. (1991) *Positive Thinking for Mental Health* (London: The Black Mental Health Group).

Freemantle, N. and Maynard, A. (1994) 'Something rotten in the state of clinical and economic evaluation', *Health Economics*, 3(2), pp. 63–8.

Freemantle, N., Song, F., Sheldon, T., Watson, P., Mason, J. and Long, A. (1993) 'Managing depression in primary care', *Quality in Health Care*, 3(2), pp. 58–62.

Freidson, E. (1970) *Profession of Medicine* (New York: Harper & Row).

Gabe, J. and Lipshitsz-Phillips, S. (1982) 'Evil necessity? The meaning of benzodiazepine use for women patients from one general practice', *Sociology of Health and Illness*, 4(2), pp. 201–11.

Gabe, J. and Thorogood, N. (1986) 'Prescribed drug use and the management of everyday life: the experiences of black and white working class women', *Sociological Review*, 34, pp. 737–72.

Gamarnikow, E. (1978) 'Sexual division of labour: the case of nursing', in A. Kuhn and A. Wolpe (eds), *Feminism and Materialism: Women and Modes of Production* (London: Routledge & Kegan Paul).

Garrett, T. (1992) *National Survey of Clinical Psychology Practitioners' Sexual Contact with Patients* (London: PROPAN).

Gask, L., Sibbald, B. and Creed, F. (1997) 'Evaluating models of working at the interface between mental health service and primary care', *British Journal of Psychiatry*, 170, pp. 6–12.

Gelinas, D. (1983) 'The persisting negative effects of incest', *Psychiatry*, 46, pp. 312–32.

Gerard, D. L. and Houston, L. G. (1953) 'Family setting and the ecology of schizophrenia', *Psychiatric Quarterly*, 27, pp. 90–101.

Giddens, A. (1991) *Modernity and Self-Identity* (Cambridge: Polity Press).

Gillam, S. and Miller, R. (1997) *A Public Health Experiment in Primary Care* (London: Kings Fund).

Ginsberg, G., Marks, I. and Waters, H. (1984) 'Cost benefit analysis of a controlled trial of nurse therapy for neuroses in primary care', *Psychological Medicine*, 14, pp. 683–90.

Glover, G., Farmer, R. and Preston, D. (1992) 'Indicators of mental hospital bed use', *Health Trends*, 22(3), pp. 111–15.

Goffman, E. (1961) *Asylums* (Harmondsworth: Penguin).

Goldberg, D. and Bridges, K. (1988) 'Somatic presentation of psychiatric illness in primary care settings', *Journal of Psychomatic Research*, 32, pp. 137–44.

Goldberg, D. and Huxley, P. (1980) *Mental Illness in the Community* (London: Tavistock).

Goldberg, D. and Huxley, P. (1992) *Common Mental Disorders* (London: Routledge).

Goldberg, D. and Morrison, S. L. (1963) 'Schizophrenia and social class', *British Journal of Psychiatry*, 109, pp. 785–802.

Goldberg, D., Sharp, D., Strathdee, G., Thornicroft, G., Mann, A., Pilgrim, D. and Rogers, A. (1993) *Developing a Strategy for a Primary Care Focus for Mental Health Services for the People of Lambeth, Southwark and Lewisham* (London: Institute of Psychiatry).

Goldie, N. (1974) 'Professional processes among three occupational groups within the mental health field', unpublished PhD, City University, London.

Goldie, N. (1977) 'The division of labour among mental health professionals – a negotiated or an imposed order?', in M. Stacey and M. Reid (eds), *Health and the Division of Labour* (London: Croom Helm).

Goodwin, S. (1992) *Community Care and the Future of Mental Health Service Provision* (Aldershot: Avebury).

Goodwin, S. (1997) *Comparative Mental Health Policy* (London: Sage).

Gough, I. (1979) *Political Economy of the Welfare State* (London: Macmillan).

Gournay, K. and Brooking, J. (1994) 'Community psychiatric nurses in primary care', *British Journal of Psychiatry*, 165, pp. 231–8.

Gove, W. (1984) 'Gender differences in mental and physical illness: the effects of fixed roles and nurturant roles', *Social Science and Medicine*, 19(2), pp. 77–91.

Gove, W. and Geerken, M. (1977) 'Response bias in surveys of mental health: an empirical investigation', *American Journal of Sociology*, 82, pp. 1289–317.

Gowler, D. and Legge, D. (1980) 'Evaluative practices as stressors in occupational settings', in C. L. Cooper and R. Payne (eds), *Current Concerns in Occupational Stress* (Chichester: Wiley).

Granshaw, L. (1989) 'Fame and fortune by means of bricks and mortar: the medical profession and specialist hospitals in Britain 1000 1910', in L. Granshaw and R. Porter (eds), *The Hospital in History* (London: Routledge).

Green, J. (1988) 'Frequent rehospitalisation and non-compliance with treatment', *Hospital and Community Psychiatry*, 39, pp. 936–66.

Greenslade, L. (1992) 'White skin, white masks: psychological distress among the Irish in Britain', in P. O'Sullivan (ed.), *The Irish in the New Communities* (Leicester: Leicester University Press).

Grohmann, R., Schmidt, L., Speiss, K. and Ruther, E. (1989) 'Agranulocytosis and significant leucopenia with neuroleptic drugs', *Psychopharmacology*, 99(109), p. 112.

Gunn, J. (1978) *Psychiatric Aspects of Imprisonment* (London: Academic Press).

Haafkens, L., Nijhof, G. and van der Poel, E. (1986) 'Mental health care and the opposition movement in the Netherlands', *Social Science and Medicine*, 22, pp. 185–92.

Habermas, J. (1971) *Toward a Rational Society* (London: Heinemann).

Hadley, T. R. and Goldman, H. (1995) 'Effect of recent health and social service policy reforms on Britain's mental health system', *British Medical Journal*, 311, pp. 1556–8.

Hagen, J. L. (1990) 'Designing service for homeless women', *Journal of Health and Social Policy*, 1, pp. 1–16.

Ham, C. (1985) *Health Policy in Britain* (London: Macmillan).

Hamid, W. (1991) 'Homeless people and community care: an assessment of the needs of homeless people', unpublished PhD thesis, University of London.

Hamilton, M. (1973) 'Psychology in society: end or ends?', *Bulletin of the British Psychological Society*, 26, pp. 185–9.

Hammer, M. (1968) 'Influence of small social networks as factors on mental hospital admission', in S. P. Spitzer and N. K. Denzin (eds), *The Mental Patient* (New York: McGraw-Hill).

Hannay, D. (1979) *Health and Lifestyles* (London: Routledge).

Hardt, R. H. and Feinhandler, S. J. (1959) 'Social class and mental hospital prognosis', *American Sociological Review*, 24, pp. 815–21.

Hare, E. (1988) 'Schizophrenia as a recent disease', *British Journal of Psychiatry*, 153, pp. 523–5.

Harrington, R. C. (1993) *Depressive Disorder in Childhood and Adolescence* (Chichester: Wiley).

Harris, E. C. and Barraclough, B. (1997) 'Suicide as an outcome for mental disorders', *British Journal of Psychiatry*, 170, pp. 205–28.

Harrison, G., Owens, D., Holton, A., Neilson, D. and Boot, D. (1988) 'A prospective study of severe mental disorder in Afro-Caribbean patients', *Psychological Medicine*, 11, pp. 289–302.

Hayes, S. C. (1998) 'Scientific practice guidelines in a political, economic and professional context', in K. S. Dobson and K. D. Craig (eds), *Empirically Supported Therapies* (London: Sage).

Hearnshaw, L. S. (1964) *A Short History of British Psychology* (London: Methuen).

Heginbotham, C. and Bosanquet, N. (1995) 'A promise of better things to come', *Health Service Journal*, 27 (July), pp. 26–7.

Heginbotham, C. and Ham, C. (1992) *Purchasing Dilemmas* (London: King's Fund College).

Hemmenki, E. (1977) 'Polypharmacy among psychiatric patients', *Acta Psychiatrica Scandinavica*, 56, pp. 347–56.

Hemsi, L. (1967) 'Psychiatric morbidity of West Indian immigrants', *Social Psychiatry*, 2, pp. 95–100.

Henderson, C., Thornicroft, G. and Glover, G. (1998) 'Inequalities in mental health', *The British Journal of Psychiatry*, 173(8), pp. 105–9.

Herman, J. L., Perrey, J. C. and vander Kolk, B. A. (1989) 'Childhood trauma in borderline personality disorder', *American Journal of Psychiatry*, 146, pp. 490–5.

Hiday, V. A., Swartz, M. S., Swanson, J. W., Borum, R. and Wagner, H. R. (1999) 'Coercion in mental health care', Unpublished paper.

Hill, R. and Leiper, R. (1992) 'Evaluation of mental health services: some quality assurance models', *International Journal of Nursing Studies*, 29, pp. 289–99.

Hirsch, S. R. (1986) 'Clinical treatment of schizophrenia', in P. B. Bradley and S. R. Hirsch (eds), *The Psychopharmacology and Treatment of Schizophrenia* (Oxford: Oxford University Press).

Hitch, P. (1981) 'Immigration and mental health: local research and social explanations', *New Community*, 9, pp. 256–62.

Hitch, P. and Clegg, P. (1980) 'Modes of referral of overseas immigrant and native-born first admissions to psychiatric hospital', *Social Science and Medicine*, 14A, pp. 369–74.

HMSO (1926) *Royal Commission on Lunacy and Mental Disorder* (London: HMSO).

HMSO (1984–5) *House of Commons Select Committee Report on Community Care* (London: HMSO).

HMSO (1986) *Mental Health Enquiry* (London: HMSO).

HMSO (1989) *Caring for People: Community Care in the Next Decade and Beyond* (London: HMSO).

HMSO (1990) (The Griffiths Report) *Community Care: Agenda for Action* (London: HMSO).

HMSO (1993) *Inpatients Formally Detained in Hospitals under the Mental Health Act 1983 and other Legislation Year ending 31st March 1990* (London: HMSO).

Hoenig, J. and Hamilton, M. (1969) *The Desegregation of the Mentally Ill* (London: Routledge & Kegan Paul).

Hoggett, B. (1990) *Mental Health Law* (London: Sweet & Maxwell).

Hogman, G. and Melzer, D. (1992) 'Talk – don't inject', *Nursing Times*, 88, pp. 62–3.

Hollingshead, A. and Redlich, R. C. (1958) *Social Class and Mental Illness* (New York: Wiley).

Horwitz, A. (1977) 'The pathways into psychiatric treatment: some differences between men and women', *Journal of Health and Social Behaviour*, 18, pp. 169–78.

240 *Bibliography*

Horwitz, A. (1983) *The Social Control of Mental Illness* (New York: Academic Press).
Hoyt, M. F. and Austad, C. S. (1992) 'Psychotherapy in a staff model maintenance organisation', *Psychotherapy*, 29, pp. 119–29.
Hughes, E. (1971) *The Sociological Eye: Selected Papers* (Chicago: Aldine Atherton).
Humphrey, M. and Haward, I. (1981) 'Sex differences in recruitment to clinical psychology', *Bulletin of the British Psychological Society*, 34, pp. 413–14.
Hunt, S. M. (1990) 'Emotional distress and bad housing', *Health and Hygiene*, 11, pp. 72–9.
Hunter, R. and MacAlpine, I. (1964) *Three Hundred Years of Psychiatry* (Oxford: Oxford University Press).
Huxley, P. (1990) *Effective Community Mental Health Services* (Aldershot: Avebury).
Hyndman, S. J. (1990) 'Housing, dampness and health among British Bengalis in East London', *Social Science and Medicine*, 30, pp. 131–41.
Ingleby, D. (1983) 'Mental health and social order', in S. Cohen and A. Scull (eds), *Social Control and the State* (Oxford: Basil Blackwell).
Islington Mental Health Forum (1989) *Fit for Consumption? Mental Health Users' Views of Treatment in Islington* (London: IMHF).
Jenkins, R. (1990) 'Towards a system of mental health outcome indicators', *British Journal of Psychiatry*, 157, pp. 500–14.
Jodelet, D. (1991) *Madness and Social Representations* (London: Harvester Wheatsheaf).
Johnstone, L. (1992) *Users and Abusers of Psychiatry* (London: Routledge).
Jones, G. and Berry, M. (1986) 'Regional Secure Units: the emerging picture', in G. Edwards (ed.), *Current Issues in Clinical Psychology* (London: Plenum Press).
Jones, K. (1960) *Mental Health and Social Policy: 1845–1959* (London: Routledge & Kegan Paul).
Jones, K. (1972) *A History of the Mental Health Services* (London: Routledge & Kegan Paul).
Jones, K. (1988) *Experience in Mental Health: Community Care and Social Policy* (London: Sage).
Jones, L. and Cochrane, R. (1981) 'Stereotypes of mental illness: a test of the labelling hypothesis', *International Journal of Social Psychiatry*, 27, pp. 99–107.
Jones, M. (1952) *Social Psychiatry* (London: Tavistock).
Jones, R. (1991) *Mental Health Act Manual*, 3rd edn (London: Sweet & Maxwell).
Judge, K. (2000) 'Testing evaluation to the limits: the case of English Health Action Zones', *Journal of Health Services Research and Policy*, 5(1), pp. 3–5.
Kane, J. M. (1985) 'Compliance issues in outpatient treatment', *Journal of Clinical Psychopharmacology*, 5, pp. 220–70.
Kay, D., Beamish, P. and Roth, M. (1964) 'Old age mental disorders in Newcastle upon Tyne, part 1, a study of prevalence', *British Journal of Psychiatry*, 110, pp. 146–8.
Kellam, A. M. P. (1987) 'The neuroleptic syndrome, so called: a survey of the world literature', *British Journal of Psychiatry*, 150, pp. 752–9.

Klassen, D. and O'Connor, W. (1987) 'Predicting violence in mental patients: cross validation of an actuarial scale', Paper presented at the annual meeting of the American Public Health Association.

Klassen, D. and O'Connor, W. (1988) 'A prospective study of predictors of violence in adult male mental patients', *Law and Human Behaviour*, 12, pp. 143–58.

Knapp, M., Hallam, A., Beecham, J. and Baines, B. (1999) 'Private, voluntary or public? Comparative cost-effectiveness in community mental health care', *Policy and Politics*, 27(1), pp. 25–43.

Kowarzik, U. and Popay, J. (1988) *That's Women's Work* (London: London Research Centre).

Lacey, R. (1991) *The MIND Complete Guide to Psychiatric Drugs* (London: Ebury Press).

Laing, R. D. (1967) *The Politics of Experience* (Harmondsworth: Penguin).

Laing, R. D. and Esterson, A. (1964) *Sanity, Madness and the Family* (Harmondsworth: Penguin).

Langer, T. S. and Michael, S. T. (1963) *Life Stress and Mental Health* (Glencoe: Free Press).

Lapouse, R., Monk, M. and Terris, W. (1956) 'The drift hypothesis and socio-economic differentials in schizophrenia', *American Journal of Public Health*, 46, pp. 968–86.

Larkin, E., Murtagh, S. and Jones, S. (1988) 'A preliminary study of violent incidents in a special hospital', *British Journal of Psychiatry*, 153, pp. 226–31.

Le Grand, J. and Robinson, R. (1981) *The Economics of Social Problems: The Market versus the State* (London: Macmillan).

Lebow, J. (1982) 'Consumer satisfaction with mental health treatment', *Psychological Bulletin*, 91(2), pp. 244–59.

Lee, J. and Gask, L. (1998) 'Past tense – future imperfect', *Health Service Journal*, 108, pp. 24–5.

Lefley, H. P. (1999) 'Mental health systems in cross-cultural context', in A. Horwitz and T. L. Scheid (eds), *A Handbook for the Study of Mental Health* (Chicago: Chicago University Press).

Leigh, C. (1994) *Everybody's Baby: Implementing Community Care for Single Homeless People* (London: CHAR).

Lemert, E. (1951) *Social Pathology* (New York: McGraw-Hill).

Lemert, E. (1967) *Human Deviance, Social Problems and Social Control* (Englewood Cliffs, NJ: Prentice-Hall).

Levine, M., Toro, P. A. and Perkins, D. V. (1993) 'Social and community interventions', *Annual Review of Psychology*, pp. 525–8.

Light, D. (1980) *Becoming Psychiatrists: The Professional Transformation of Self* (Chicago: W. Norton).

Light, D. (1985) 'Professional training and the future of psychiatry', in P. Brown (ed.), *Mental Health Care and Social Policy* (Boston, Massachusetts: Routledge & Kegan Paul).

Link, B. and Stueve, A. (1998) Editorial, *Archives of General Psychiatry*, 55, pp. 1–3.

Little, J. (1990) 'Can health be promoted?', in J. Martin and L. McQueen (eds), *Readings for a New Public Health* (Edinburgh: Edinburgh University Press).

Littlewood, R. and Cross, S. (1980) 'Ethnic minorities and psychiatric services', *Sociology of Health and Illness*, 2, pp. 194–201.

Littlewood, R. and Lipsedge, M. (1982) *Aliens and Alienists* (Harmondsworth: Penguin).

Lomax, M. (1921) *Experiences of an Asylum Doctor, with Suggestions for Asylum and Lunacy Law Reform* (London: George Allen & Unwin).

Lyon, M. (1996) 'C. Wright Mills meets Prozac: the relevance of social emotion to the sociology of health and illness', *Health and the Sociology of Emotions*, Sociology of Health and Illness Monograph, edited by V. James and J. Gabe (Oxford: British Sociology Association).

Macdonald, G. and O'Hara, K. (1998) *Ten Elements of Mental Health, its Promotion and Demotion: Implications for Practice* (Glasgow: Society of Health Education and Health Promotion Specialists).

Main, T. (1957) 'The ailment', *British Journal of Medical Psychology*, 30, p. 29.

Maloy, K. (1992) *Critiquing the Empirical Evidence: Does Involuntary Outpatient Commitment Work?* (Washington DC: Mental Health Policy Center).

Mangen, S. (1994) 'Continuing care: an emerging issue in European health policy', *International Journal of Social Psychiatry*, 40(4), pp. 235–45.

Mangen, S., Paykel, E., Griffith, J., Burchell, A. and Mancini, P. (1983) 'Cost effectiveness of community psychiatric nurse or outpatient psychiatrist care of neurotic patients', *Psychological Medicine*, 13, pp. 401–16.

Manthorpe, J. (1994) 'The family and informal care', in N. Malin (ed.), *Implementing Community Care* (Buckingham: Open University Press).

Marks, I. (1992) 'Innovations in mental health care', *British Journal of Psychiatry*, 160, pp. 589–97.

Marmor, T. R. (1973) *The Politics of Medicare* (Chicago: Aldine).

Marshall, M., Bond, G. and Stein, A. (1999) 'The PRiSM psychosis study: design limitations, questionable conclusions', *British Journal of Psychiatry*, 175, pp. 501–3.

Martin, D. and Lyon, P. (1984) 'Lesbian women and mental health policy', in L. E. Walker (ed.), *Women and Mental Health Policy* (London: Sage).

Martin, J. P. (1985) *Hospitals in Trouble* (Oxford: Basil Blackwell).

Masson, J. (1988) *Against Therapy* (London: HarperCollins).

Mayer, J. and Timms, N. (1970) *The Client Speaks* (London: Routledge & Kegan Paul).

McGovern, D. and Cope, R. (1987) 'The compulsory detention of males of different ethnic groups with special reference to offender patients', *British Journal of Psychiatry*, 150, pp. 505–12.

McIntyre, K., Farrell, M. and David, A. (1989) 'What do psychiatric inpatients really want?', *British Medical Journal*, 298, pp. 159–60.

McMillan, I. (1995) 'Reviewing the review', *Nursing Times*, 91 (3 May), p. 18.

Means, R. and Smith, R. (1994) *Community Care: Policy and Practice* (London: Macmillan).

Mechanic, D. (1969) *Mental Health and Social Policy* (Englewood Cliffs, NJ: Prentice-Hall).

Medawar, C. (1992) *Power and Dependence* (London: Social Audit).

Meltzer, H., Baljit, G. and Petticrew, M. (1994) *The Prevalance of Psychiatric Morbidity among Adults aged 16–64 Living in Private Households in Great Britain*, Bulletin No. 1 (London: OPCS Social Survey Division).

Mental Health Foundation (1994) *Creating Community Care* (London: Mental Health Foundation).

Miller, J. (1991) 'The doctor's dilemma: Miller on Madness, *OpenMind*, 49, February, p. 31.

Miller, P. (1986) 'Critiques of psychiatry and critical sociologies of madness', in P. Miller and N. Rose (eds), *The Power of Psychiatry* (Cambridge: Polity Press).

Miller, P. and Rose, N. (1988) 'The Tavistock programme: the government of subjectivity and social life', *Sociology*, 22(2), pp. 171–92.

Mills, E. (1962) *Living with Mental Illness* (London: Institute of Community Studies/Routledge & Kegan Paul).

Mills, M. (1992) *SHANTI – A Consumer-Based Approach to Planning Mental Health Services for Women* (London: SHANTI Women's Counselling Services).

Ministry of Health (1963) *Health and Welfare: the Development of Community Care* (London: HMSO).

Mirowsky, J. and Ross, C. (1989) 'Psychiatric diagnosis as reified measurement', *Journal of Health and Social Behaviour*, 30, pp. 11–25.

Monahan, J. (1973) 'The psychiatrization of criminal behaviour: a reply', *Hospital and Community Psychiatry*, 24(2), pp. 105–7.

Monahan, J. (1981) *Predicting Violent Behaviour* (Beverly Hills, California: Sage).

Monahan, J. (1992) 'Mental disorder and violent behaviour perceptions and evidence', *American Psychologist*, 47(4), pp. 511–21.

Monahan, J. and Steadman, H. J. (eds) (1994) *Violence and Mental Disorder: Developments in Risk Assessment* (Chicago: Chicago University Press).

Morris, B. S. (1949) 'Officer selection in the British Army', *Occupational Psychology*, 23, pp. 219–34.

Murphy, E. (1993) 'Mental illness and community care', paper presented at the Conference of the Association of Social Service Directors, Solihull, October.

Myers, J. (1974) 'Social class, life events and psychiatric symptoms: a longitudinal study', in B. S. Dohrenwend and B. P. Dohrenwend (eds), *Stressful Life Events: Their Nature and Effects* (New York: Wiley).

Myers, J. (1975) 'Life events, social integration and psychiatric symptomatology', *Journal of Health and Social Behaviour*, 16, pp. 121–7.

Myers, J. and Bean, L. (1968) *A Decade Later: A Follow Up of Social Class and Mental Illness* (New York: Wiley).

Netten, A. and Dennet, J. (1997) *Unit Costs of Health and Social Care* (Canterbury: University of Kent PSSRU).

Newton, J. (1988) *Preventing Mental Illness* (London: Routledge).

NHSME (1994) *Introduction of Supervision Registers for Mentally Ill People from 1 April 1994* (Leeds: DH).

NHSME (1994) *Guidance on the Discharge of Mentally Disordered People and Their Continuing Care in the Community* (HSG (94)27) (London: DH).

NHSME Mental Health Task Force (1994) *Black Mental Health – A Dialogue for Change* (London: DH).

Nicolson, P. (1989) 'Counselling women with post-natal depression', *Counselling Psychology Quarterly*, 2, pp. 123–32.

Nicolson, P. (1992) 'Gender issues in the organisation of clinical psychology', in J. Ussher and P. Nicolson (eds), *Gender Issues in Clinical Psychology* (London: Routledge).

Nilbert, D., Cooper, S. and Crossmaker, M. (1989) 'Assaults against residents of a psychiatric institution: residents' history of abuse', *Journal of Interpersonal Violence*, 4(3), pp. 342–9.

Norris, M. (1984) *Integration of Special Hospital Patients into the Community* (Aldershot: Gower).

Nuffield Provincial Hospitals Trust (1994) *Housing, Homelessness and Health* (London: Nuffield Provincial Hospitals Trust).

O'Brien, J. (1992) 'Closing the asylums: where do all the former long-stay patients go?', *Health Trends*, 24(3), pp. 88–90.

Offe, C. (1984) *Contradictions of the Welfare State* (London: Hutchinson).

Office for National Statistics (1997) *1995 Mortality Statistics: Cause*, England and Wales Series DH2 no 22 (London: HMSO).

Olfsen, M. (1990) 'Assertive community treatment: an evaluation of the experimental evidence', *Hospital and Community Psychiatry*, 41, pp. 634–41.

Oliver, M. (1987) *The Politics of Disablement* (London: Macmillan).

Oliver, J., Huxley, P., Bridges, K. and Mohamad, H. (1996) *Quality of Life and Mental Health Services* (London: Routledge).

Onyett, S., Heppleston, T. and Bushnell, D. (1994a) 'A national survey of community mental health team structure and process', *Journal of Mental Health*, 3, pp. 175–94.

Onyett, S., Heppleston, T. and Bushnell, D. (1994b) 'Job satisfaction and burnout in community mental health team members', unpublished paper.

Onyett, S., Standen, R. and Peck, E. (1997) 'The challenge of managing community mental health teams', *Health and Social Care in the Community*, 5, pp. 40–7.

OPCS (1977) *Mortality Statistics* (London: HMSO).

OPCS (1994) *National Psychiatric Morbidity Survey* (London: HMSO).

Oppenheimer, M. (1975) 'The proletarianisation of the professional', *Sociological Review Monograph*, 20.

Orwell, G. (1986) *Down and Out in Paris and London* (Harmondsworth: Penguin).

Ostamo, A. and Lonnqvist, J. (1992) 'Parasuicide rates by gender in Helsinki, 1988–91', poster paper at Joint Conference of the British Sociological Association Medical Sociology Group and the European Society of Medical Sociology (Edinburgh).

Palmer, G. (1978) 'Social and political determinants of changes in health care financing and delivery', in A. Graycar (ed.), *Perspectives in Australian Social Policy* (Melbourne: Macmillan).

Palmer, G. and Short, S. (1989) *Health Care and Public Policy: An Australian Analysis* (Melbourne: Macmillan).

Parker, E. (1985) 'The development of secure provision', in L. Gostin (ed.), *Secure Provision* (London: Tavistock).

Parker, I., Georgaca, E., Harper, D., McLaughlin, T. and Stowell-Smith, M., (1995) *Deconstructing Psychopathology* (London: Sage).

Parker, M. M. (1992) 'Post-modern organisations or post-modern organisational theory?', *Organisation Studies*, 13(1), pp. 1–19.

Parkhouse, J. (1991) *Doctors' Careers: Aims and Experiences of Medical Graduates* (London: Routledge).

Parry, G. (1992) 'Improving psychotherapy services: applications of research, audit and evaluation', *British Journal of Clinical Psychology*, 31, pp. 3–19.

Parry, N. and Parry, G. (1977) 'Professionalism and unionism: aspects of class conflicts in the National Health Service', *Sociological Review*, 25(4), pp. 823–40.

Patmore, C. and Weaver, T. (1991) *Community Mental Health Centres: Lessons for Planners and Managers* (London: Good Practices in Mental Health).

Pavis, S., Masters, H., Cunningham-Burley, S. (1996) *Lay Concepts of Positive Mental Health and How it can be Maintained* (Edinburgh: Department of Public Health Sciences, University of Edinburgh).

Paykel, E. (1990) 'Innovations in mental health care in the primary care system', in I. Marks and R. Scott (eds), *Mental Health Care Delivery* (Cambridge: Cambridge University Press).

Peay, J. (1989) *Tribunals on Trial: A Study of Decision-Making under the Mental Health Act 1983* (Oxford: Oxford University Press).

Peck, E. and Cockburn, M. (1993) 'Comparative costs of adult acute psychiatric services', *Psychiatric Bulletin*, 17, pp. 79–81.

Perring, C., Twigg, J. and Atkin, K. (1990) *Families Caring for People Diagnosed as Mentally Ill* (London: HMSO).

Philo, G., Secker, J. and Platt, S. (1996) 'Media Images of mental distress', in T. Heller *et al.* (eds), *Mental Health Matters: A Reader* (Basingstoke: Macmillan).

Pilgrim, D. (1997) 'Some reflections on "quality" and "mental health"', *Journal of Mental Health*, 6(6), pp. 567–76.

Pilgrim. D. (1999) 'Making the best of clinical governance', *Journal of Mental Health*, 8(1), pp. 1–2.

Pilgrim, D. and Bentall, R. P. (1999) 'The medicalisation of misery: a critical realist analysis of the concept of depression', *Journal of Mental Health* 8(3), pp. 261–74.

Pilgrim, D. and Guinan, P. (1999) 'From mitigation to culpability: re-thinking the evidence about therapist sexual abuse', *European Journal of Psychotherapy, Counselling and Health*, 2(2), pp. 153–68.

Pilgrim, D. and Hoser, B. (1999) *Users' and carers' views of mental health services in the NW of England* (Warrington: NHSE)

Pilgrim, D. and Rogers, A. (1993) *A Sociology of Mental Health and Illness* (Buckingham: Open University Press).

Pilgrim, D. and Rogers, A. (1994) 'Something old something new: sociology and the organisation of psychiatry', *Sociology*, 28(2), pp. 521–38.

Pilgrim, D. and Rogers, A. (1998) 'Two notions of note in mental health debates', in T. Heller *et al.* (eds), *Mental Health Matters* (Basingstoke: Macmillan).

Pilgrim, D. and Rogers, A. (1999) 'Mental health policy and the politics of mental health: a three tier analytical framework', *Policy and Politics*, 27(1), pp. 13–24.

Pilgrim, D. and Rogers A. (1999a) *A Sociology of Mental Health and Illness* (2nd Edition) (Buckingham: Open University Press).

Pilgrim, D., Rogers, A., Clarke, S. and Clark, W. (1997) 'Entering psychological treatment: decision making factors for GPs and service users', *Journal of Interprofessional Care*, 11(3), pp. 313–23.

Pilgrim, D. and Treacher, A. (1992) *Clinical Psychology Observed* (London: Routledge).

Popay, J. (1992) '"My health is all right, but I'm just tired all the time": women's experience of ill health', in H. Roberts (ed.), *Women's Health Matters* (London: Routledge).

Porter, R. (1987) *Mind Forged Manacles* (Harmondsworth: Penguin).

Prior, D., Stewart, J. and Walsh, K. (1995) *Citizenship: Rights, Community and Participation* (London: Pitman).

Prior, L. (1991) 'Mind, Body and Behaviour. Theorisation of Madness and the Organisation of Therapy', *Sociology*, 25(3) pp. 403–22.

Prior, P. (1993) *Mental Health and Politics in Northern Ireland* (Aldershot: Avebury).

Privy Council Office (1947) *The Work of Psychology and Psychologists in the Services: Report of an Expert Committee* (London: HMSO).

Punch, M. (1979) 'The secret social service', in S. Holdaway (ed.), *The British Police* (London: Edward Arnold).

Rack, P. (1982) *Race, Culture and Mental Disorder* (London: Tavistock).

Ramon, S. (1985) *Psychiatry in Britain: Meaning and Policy* (London: Gower).

Ramon, S. (1986) 'The category of psychopathy: its professional and social context in Britain', in P. Miller and N. Rose (eds), *The Power of Psychiatry* (Cambridge: Polity Press).

Ramon, S. (ed.) (1991) *Beyond Community Care: Normalisation and Integration Work* (London: Macmillan).

Read, J. and Wallcraft, J. (1992) *Guidelines for Empowering Users of Mental Health Services* (Banstead: COHSE).

Ritchie, L., Dick, D. and Lingham, R. (1994) *The Report of the Inquiry into the Care and Treatment of Christopher Clunis* (London: HMSO).

Rochefort, D. (1988) 'Policy making cycles in mental health: critical examination of a conceptual model', *Journal of Health Politics, Policy and Law*, 13(1), pp. 129–51.

Rogers, A. (1990) 'Policing mental disorder: controversies, myths and realities', *Social Policy and Administration*, 24(3), pp. 226–37.

Rogers, A. (1993) 'Police and psychiatrists', *Social Policy and Administration*, 27(1), pp. 33–58.

Rogers, A. and Elliott, H. (1997) *Primary Care: Understanding Health Need and Demand* (Alingdon: Radcliffe Medical Press).

Rogers, A. and Pilgrim, D. (1986) 'Mental Health reforms: contrasts between Britain and Italy', *Free Associations*, 6, pp. 65–79.

Rogers, A. and Pilgrim, D. (1989) 'Citizenship and mental health', *Critical Social Policy*, 26, pp. 25–32.

Rogers, A. and Pilgrim, D. (1991) '"Pulling down churches": accounting for the British mental health users' movement', *Sociology of Health and Illness*, 13(2), pp. 129–48.

Rogers, A. and Pilgrim, D. (1993) 'Service users' views of psychiatric treatments', *Sociology of Health and Illness*, 15(5), pp. 612–31.

Rogers, A. and Pilgrim, D. (1997) 'The contribution of lay knowledge to the understanding and promotion of mental health', *Journal of Mental Health*, 6(1), pp. 23–5.

Rogers, A., Pilgrim, D. and Lacey, R. (1993) *Experiencing Psychiatry: Users' Views of Services* (London: Macmillan).

Rogers, A., Pilgrim, D. and Latham, M. (1996) *Understanding and Promoting*

Mental Health: a Study of Familial Views and Conduct in their Social Contexts (London: Health Education Authority).

Rogers, A. and Rassaby, E. (1986) 'Have you opted out? Social work under the Mental Health Act', *Community Care*, 696, pp. 20–2.

Rogers, A., *et al.* (1997) 'Experiencing depression, experiencing, the depressed', *Journal of Mental Health*.

Rose, N. (1986) 'Law, rights and psychiatry', in P. Miller and N. Rose (eds), *The Power of Psychiatry* (Cambridge: Polity Press).

Rose, N. (1990) *Governing the Soul* (London: Routledge).

Rose, S. M., Peabody, C. G. and Stratigeas, B. (1991) 'Undetected abuse among intensive case management clients', *Hospital and Community Psychiatry*, 42(5), pp. 235–50.

Rosen, G. (1968) *Madness in Society* (New York: Harper & Row).

Rosen, G. (1979) 'The evolution of scientific medicine', in H. Freeman, S. Levine and L. Reeder (eds), *Handbook of Medical Sociology* (Englewood Cliffs, NJ: Prentice-Hall).

Rosenhan, D. L. (1973) 'On being sane in insane places', *Science*, 179, pp. 250–8.

Roth, M. (1973) 'Psychiatry and its critics', *British Journal of Psychiatry*, 122, p. 374.

Rothblum, E. D. (1990) 'Depression among lesbians: an invisible and unresearched phenomenon', *Journal of Gay and Lesbian Psychotherapy*, 1, pp. 67–87.

Royal College of Psychiatrists (Scottish Division) (1973) *The Future of Psychiatric Services in Scotland* (London: Royal College of Psychiatrists).

Royal Commission on National Health Insurance (1926) *Report for the Ministry of Health* (London: Ministry of Health).

Rwgellera, G. G. C. (1977) 'Psychiatric morbidity among West Africans and West Indians living in London', *Psychological Medicine*, 7, pp. 317–29.

Sainsbury Centre (1998) *Acute Problems: A Survey of the Quality of Care in Acute Psychiatric Wards* (London: Sainsbury Centre for Mental Health).

Saks, M. (1983) 'Removing the blinkers? A critique of recent contributions to the sociology of the professions', *The Sociological Review*, 2, pp. 1–21.

Samele, C. (1993) 'The impact of law 180 on women carers', unpublished PhD thesis, University of Kent.

Samson, C. (1992) 'Confusing symbolic event with reality: the case of community mental health in the USA', paper presented at the Conference of the British Sociological Association Medical Sociology Group and the European Society of Medical Sociology.

Samson, C. (1995) 'The fracturing of medical dominance in British Psychiatry', *Sociology of Health and Illness*, 17(2), pp. 245–69.

Sankey Committee on Voluntary Hospitals (1937) Report for the *British Hospitals Association* (London: BHA).

Sashidharan, S. P. (1986) 'Ideology and politics in transcultural psychiatry', in J. L. Cox (ed.), *Transcultural Psychiatry* (London: Croom Helm).

Sayce, L. (1989) 'Community mental health centres – rhetoric and reality', in A. Brackx and C. Grimshaw (eds), *Mental Health Care in Crisis* (London: Pluto).

Sayce, L. (1990) 'Care reforms dislocated', *OpenMind*, 46, p. 5.

Sayce, L. (2000) *From Psychiatric Patient to Citizen* (London: Macmillan).

Scheff, T. (1966) *Being Mentally Ill: A Sociological Theory* (Chicago: Aldine).

Scott, J., Normanton, M. and McKenna, J. (1990) 'Developing a community orientated mental health service', *Psychiatric Bulletin*, 16, pp. 150–2.

Scott, R. D. (1973) 'The treatment barrier, part V', *British Journal of Medical Psychology*, 46, pp. 45–53.

Scull, A. (1977) *Decarceration: Community Treatment and the Deviant – A Radical View* (Englewood Cliffs, NJ: Prentice-Hall).

Scull, A. (1979) *Museums of Madness* (Harmondsworth: Penguin).

Seagar, C. P. (1991) 'Management of district psychiatric services without a mental hospital', in P. Hall and I. Brockington (eds), *The Closure of Mental Hospitals* (London: Gaskell/Royal College of Psychiatrists).

Sedgwick, P. (1982) *Psychopolitics* (London: Pluto Press).

Shaikh, S. (1985) 'Cross-cultural comparison, psychiatric admissions of Asian and indigenous patients in Leicestershire', *International Journal of Social Psychiatry*, 31, pp. 3–11.

Sheppard, M. (1990) 'Social work and psychiatric nursing', in P. Abbott and C. Wallace (eds), *The Sociology of the Caring Professions* (London: Falmer Press).

Sheppard, M. (1991) 'General practice, social work and mental health sections: the social control of women', *British Journal of Social Work*, 21, pp. 663–83.

Showalter, E. (1985) *The Female Malady* (London: Virago).

Sibbald, B., Addington-Hall, J., Brennerman, D. and Freeling, P. (1993) 'Counsellors in English and Welsh General Practices: their nature and distribution', *British Medical Journal*, 302, pp. 28–33.

Sibbald, B., Addington-Hall, J., Brenneman, D. and Freeling, P. (1993) in the *British Medical Journal*, 307, pp. 544–6.

Skultans, V. (1979) *English Madness: Ideas on Insanity, 1580–1890* (London: Routledge & Kegan Paul).

Snow, D., Baker, S., Anderson, L. and Martin, M. (1986) 'The myth of pervasive mental illness amongst the homeless', *Social Problems*, 33, pp. 407–23.

Spicker, S. (1993) 'Going off the dole: a prudential and ethical critique of the health fare State', *Health Care Analysis*, 1, pp. 11–16.

Steadman, H., Monahan, J., Applebaum, P., Grisso, T., Milvey, E., Roth, L., Clark Robbins, P. and Klassen, D. (1994) 'Designing a new generation of risk assessment research', in J. Monahan and H. Steadman (eds), *Violence and Mental Disorder: Developments in Risk Assessment* (Chicago: University of Chicago Press).

Stein, L. and Test, M. (1980) 'Alternative to mental hospital treatment', *Archives of General Hospital Psychiatry*, 37, pp. 392–7.

Stewart, M. B., Browne, B., Weston, W., McWhinney, I., McWilliam, C. and Freeman, T. (1995) *Patient Centred Medicine: Transforming the Clinical Method* (London: Sage).

Stone, M. (1985) 'Shellshock and the psychologists', in W. F. Bynum, R. Porter and M. Shepherd (eds), *The Anatomy of Madness*, Vol. 2 (London: Tavistock).

Strathdee, G. and Williams, P. (1984) 'A survey of psychiatrists in primary care: the silent growth of a new service', *Journal of the Royal College of General Practitioners*, 34, pp. 615–18.

Swartz, M. S., Swanson, J. W., Wagner, H. R., Burns, B. J., Hiday, V. A. and Borum, R. (1999) 'Can involuntary outpatient commitment reduce hospital recidivism?: Findings from a randomized trial with severely mentally ill individuals', *American Journal of Psychiatry*, 156(12), pp. 1968–75.

Szasz, T. S. (1961) 'The uses of naming and the origin of the myth of mental illness', *American Psychologist*, 16, pp. 59–65.

Szasz, T. S. (1962) *The Myth of Mental Illness* (New York: Harper).

Szasz, T. S. (1963) *Law, Liberty and Psychiatry* (New York: Macmillan).

Szasz, T. S. (1971) *The Manufacture of Madness* (London: Routledge & Kegan Paul).

Taylor, P. L. and Gunn, J. (1984) 'Violence and psychosis 1: risk of violence among psychotic men', *British Medical Journal*, 288, pp. 1945–9.

Teasdale, K. (1987) 'Stigma and psychiatric day care', *Journal of Advanced Nursing*, 12, pp. 339–46.

Teplin, L. A. (ed.) (1984) *Mental Health and Criminal Justice* (New York: Sage).

Thompson, D. (1987) 'Coalitions and conflict in the National Health Service: some implications for general management', *Sociology of Health and Illness*, 9(2), pp. 127–53.

Thornicroft, G. and Strathdee, G. (1991) 'Mental Health', *British Medical Journal*, 17 August, pp. 410–12.

Thornicroft G., Brewin, C. and Wing, J. (1992) *Measuring Mental Health Needs* (London: Gaskell).

Titley, M., Watson, G. and Williams, J. (1992) 'Working women, including older women, in the mental health services', paper presented at the London Conference of the British Psychological Society.

Titmuss, R. (1958) *Essays on the Welfare State* (London: George Allen & Unwin).

Titmuss, R. (1968) *Commitment to Welfare* (London: George Allen & Unwin).

Tomes, N. (1988) 'The great restraint controversy: a comparative perspective on Anglo-American psychiatry in the nineteenth century', in W. Bynum, R. Porter and M. Shepherd (eds), *The Anatomy of Madness: Essays in the History of Madness* (London: Routledge).

Tomlinson, D. (1991) *Utopia, Community Care and the Retreat from the Asylums* (Buckingham: Open University Press).

Trent Regional Health Authority (1992) *Trent Health GP Fundholding Initiative Price List: Final Version 1992/3* (Nottingham: Trent RHA).

Tudor, K. (1991) 'One step back, two steps forward: community care and mental health', *Critical Social Policy*, 30, pp. 5–23.

Turner, B. S. (1990) 'The interdisciplinary curriculum: from social medicine to post-modernism', *Sociology of Health and Illness*, 12(1), pp. 1–23.

Turner-Crowson, J. (1993) *Reshaping Mental Health Services* (London: King's Fund Institute).

Veblen, T. (1925) *The Theory of the Leisure Class* (London: Routledge).

Vernon, P. E. and Parry, J. B. (1949) *Personnel Selection in the British Forces* (London: London University Press).

Wagenfeld, M. (1983) 'Primary prevention and public mental health policy', *Journal of Public Health Policy*, 4(2), pp. 168–80.

Walker, N. and McCabe, S. (1973) *Crime and Insanity in England*, Vol. 1 (Edinburgh: Edinburgh University Press).

Warner, R. (1985) *Recovery from Schizophrenia: Psychiatry and Political Economy* (London: Routledge).
Webster, C. (1988) *The Health Services since the War*, Vol. 1 (London: HMSO).
Weissman, M. and Klerman, G. (1978) 'Epidemiology of mental disorder: emerging trends in the US', *Archives of General Psychiatry*, 35, pp. 705–12.
Weller, B. and Weller, M. (1989) 'Prison – the psychiatric dumping ground', *New Law Journal*, 6 October, p. 1333.
Weller, M. (1985) 'Friern Hospital: where have all the patients gone?', *The Lancet*, 1, pp. 569–70.
Westermeyer, J. and Kroll, J. (1978) 'Violence and mental illness in a peasant society: characteristics of violent behaviours and "folk" use of restraints', *British Journal of Psychiatry*, 133, pp. 529–41.
Whiteley, J. (1955) "Down and Out in London": mental illness in the lower social groups', *The Lancet*, 1, pp. 553–4.
Whitton, A., Warner, R. and Appleby, L. (1996) 'The pathway to care in post natal depression: women's attitudes to post natal depression and its treatment', *British Journal of General Practice*, 46(408), pp. 427–8.
WHO Regional Office for Europe (1985) *Targets for Health for All* (Copenhagen: WHO).
Wilkinson, R. G. (1996) *Unhealthy Societies: The Afflictions of Inequality* (London: Routledge).
Williams, L., Watson, G., Smith, H., Copperman, J. and Wood, D. (1993) *Purchasing Effective Mental Health Services for Women: A Framework for Action* (Canterbury: University of Kent).
Williams, P., Tarnopolosky, A., Hand, D. and Shepherd, M. (1986) 'Minor psychiatric morbidity and general practice consultations: the West London Survey', *Psychological Medicine Monograph Supplement*, 9.
Williamson, C. (1993) *Whose Standards?* (Buckingham: Open University Press).
Wing, L. K. (ed.) (1985) *Health Service Planning and Research: Contributions of Case Registers* (London: Gaskell).
Wing, J., Curtiss, C. and Beevor, M. (1996) *Health of the Nation Scales for Mental Health* (London: Royal College of Psychiatrists).
Wing, L. K. and Freudenberg, R. K. (1961) 'The response of severely ill chronic schizophrenic patients to social stimulation', *American Journal of Psychiatry*, 118, p. 311.
Winnicott, D. W. (1958) *Collected Works* (London: Hogarth Press).
Wolfe, J. and Tumim, S. (1990) *Prison Disturbances 1990* (The Tumim Report) Cmnd 1456 (London: HMSO).
Wolfensberger, W. (ed.) (1972) *Normalisation: The Principle of Normalisation in Human Services* (Toronto: National Institue for Medical Research).
Wootton, B. (1959) *Social and Science and Social Pathology* (London: George Allen & Unwin).

Index

CTOs, 220
'dissident' psychiatrists, 108
financing of mental health
  services, 209
mental health law, 17, 197
mental health service movement,
  110
mental health services, 8
'mental health status' of homeless
  people, 36
New Right thinkers, 71
primary prevention (case study),
  130–3
primary prevention approach,
  140–1
'privatised system of welfare', 8
research on therapist variables, 188
self-harm, 197
sterilisation of patients, 14
strong reaction against asylums
  (1960s, 1970s), 70
use of psychiatric services to
  detain sane people, 107
universalism, 8
universities, 90, 127
urban regeneration, 140
urbanisation, 44, 47
USSR, 107
Utah, 209
utopianism, 159

Victorians: lunacy policy, 46
  see also asylums
violence, 32, 50–1, 162, 169, 180,
  197, 205, 207, 225, 226
assault, 91
Clunis case, 162–4
domestic, 200
murder, 10, 30
potential, 215
sexual and non-sexual, 198
against women, 200
  see also abuse; suicide
vocational guidance, 126
voluntary
boarder system, 55
hospital movement, 41–2
organisations, 67
relationships, 176–7

sector, 75, 83–4, 113, 212, 214,
  219, 225
services, 69
vulnerability, 209

wage labour, [43–]44
Wagenfeld, M., 133
Wales
CPA 'does not apply' in, 164
National Assembly, x
PCGs/PCTs, 150
Wallace, Marjorie, 224
Warner, R., 11, 138
wealth: mitigatory factor, 36
Weaver, T., *see* Patmore, C.
Weber, Max (1864–1920), 12
welfare
economics, 7
paternalism, 71
restructuring, 78
spending (1970s and after), 73
welfare state, 129
crisis (1970s) of, 70
impact of restructuring (1980s), 71
'mixed economy', 8, 69
pre-1979, 69
welfare states, 11, 16
well-being, 208
Western Europe, 16
White Papers
*Better Services for the Mentally
  Ill* (1975), 159–60
Caring for People (1989), 81
on health (1944), 59
*New NHS: Modern and
  Dependable* (1997), 150
'White Paper 10', 90
widowhood, 132
Williams, L., *et al.* (1993), 200
Williamson, C., 19–20, 118–20
Wing, J.K., *see* Brown, G. W.
women, 52, 186, 204
abuse of, 201
black, 200
depression, [68–]69, 137, 201
discrimination against, [105–]106,
  200
ethnic minority, 200
factory working hours, 51